GETTING AHEAD IN MEDICINE

A GUIDE TO PERSONAL SKILLS FOR DOCTORS

GETTING AHEAD IN MEDICINE

A GUIDE TO PERSONAL SKILLS FOR DOCTORS

C.J.H. Johnson, C.R. Hall

*Anaesthetic Department, Southmead Hospital,
Bristol, UK*

and

F.C. Forrest

*Sir Humphry Davy Department of Anaesthesia,
Bristol Royal Infirmary,
Bristol, UK*

*β*IOS
SCIENTIFIC
PUBLISHERS

© BIOS Scientific Publishers Limited, 1998

First published 1998

A CIP catalogue record for this book is available from the British Library.

ISBN 1 859960 21 9

BIOS Scientific Publishers Ltd
9 Newtec Place, Magdalen Road, Oxford OX4 1RE, UK
Tel. +44 (0) 1865 726286. Fax +44 (0) 1865 246823
World Wide Web home page: http://www.BIOS.co.uk/

DISTRIBUTORS

Australia and New Zealand
    Blackwell Science Asia
    54 University Street
    Carlton, South Victoria 3053

India
    Viva Books Private Limited
    4325/3 Ansari Road, Daryaganj
    New Delhi 110002

Singapore and South East Asia
    Toppan Company (S) PTE Ltd
    38 Liu Fang Road, Jurong
    Singapore 2262

USA and Canada
    BIOS Scientific Publishers
    PO Box 605, Herndon
    VA 20172-0605

Important Note from the Publisher
The information contained within this book was obtained by BIOS Scientific Publishers Ltd from sources believed by us to be reliable. However, while every effort has been made to ensure its accuracy, no responsibility for loss or injury whatsoever occasioned to any person acting or refraining from action as a result of information contained herein can be accepted by the authors or publishers.

The reader should remember that medicine is a constantly evolving science and while the authors and publishers have ensured that all dosages, applications and practices are based on current indications, there may be specific practices which differ between communities. You should always follow the guidelines laid down by the manufacturers of specific products and the relevant authorities in the country in which you are practising.

Typeset by Creative Associates, Oxford, UK.
Printed by Biddles Ltd, Guildford, UK.
Cover Design by Designers and Partners, Oxford, UK.

CONTENTS

(The logos denote topics of practical interest at the skill levels shown.)

ABBREVIATIONS

A-V	audio visual (aid)
ACME	Advisory Committee on Medical Establishments
AGMETS	Advisory Group on Medical and Dental Education, Training and Staffing (England and Wales)
AOB	any other business (in a committee meeting)
APACHE	acute physiology age chronic health evaluation
ARR	absolute risk reduction
BIT	binary digit
BMJ	*British Medical Journal*
CAL	computer-aided learning
CCST	Certificate of Completion of Specialist Training
CD-ROM	compact disk-read only memory
CEPOD	confidential enquiry into peri-operative deaths
CME	continuing medical education
CPC	clinico-pathological conference
CPU	central processing unit (of a computer)
CV	curriculum vitae
dpi	dots per inch (computer screen or printer definition)
DVD	digital versatile disk
EEC	European Economic Community
EPR	electronic patient record
GMC	General Medical Council (of the United Kingdom)
GP	general practitioner (family doctor)
HMO	health maintenance organization
IT	information technology
LREC	Local Research Ethics Committee
M&M	morbidity and mortality (meeting)
MAAG	medical audit advisory group
MB	megabyte (one million bytes — a unit of computer memory)
MCQ	multiple choice questionnaire
MRC	Medical Research Council
MREC	Multicentre Research Ethics Committee
NCEPOD	National Confidential Enquiry into Peri-operative Deaths
NHD	notional half day (unit of workload in consultant contract)
NHS	National Health Service (of the United Kingdom)
NNT	number needed to treat
OHT	overhead transparency
OMR	optical mark reader
OSCE	objective structured clinical examination
PAS	patient administration system
PC	personal computer
PRHO	pre-registration house officer
POWAR	place of work accredited representative
quango	quasi-autonomous non-governmental organization
RAM	random access memory (of a computer)
RRR	relative risk reduction
SHO	Senior House Officer
SWOT	Strengths/Weaknesses/Opportunities/Threats — a management tool
SpR	Specialist Registrar
TRISS	trauma injury scoring system
WORM	write-once read-many (a form of computer memory)

USING THIS BOOK

This book consists of 14 chapters, each sub-divided into sections. Each chapter begins with a set of objectives. Some sections are practical guides to completing a task; others provide background information designed to make you think more deeply about a topic, or enable you to answer an interview question. At the end of the book we have included a set of skill exercises to emphasize the points mentioned in the text and to enable you to assess your progress.

You could read this book from beginning to end, but we think that you would rapidly become saturated with information. Instead we recommend that you select the sections that are relevant to you at each stage in your career. To help you select which topics to read about, we have divided the book into four skill levels:

Level 1   Appropriate for student and pre-registration house officer years
Level 2   Required as a senior house officer
Level 3   Learned as a registrar
Level 4   Acquired as an experienced registrar or consultant

You will find these categories in the boxes overleaf. Practical information relating to these skill levels is also indicated in the Contents list.

We have been anxious to keep this book compact, so there are some large topics that we have deliberately covered superficially. When appropriate, we have included references to other texts which we think will enable the interested reader to explore a subject in greater detail.

We know from the comments we received from those who read drafts of this book that doctors hold disparate views about, for instance, the best way to give a case presentation or produce a CV. We think that the advice we offer is sensible, but would always recommend that you also seek advice from seniors in your own region.

PREFACE

In the past, medical training has produced doctors who were skilled clinicians and researchers, but nowadays doctors are expected to acquire many additional skills. Trainees are expected to be able to work efficiently, communicate, teach, understand the principles of audit and evidence-based medicine, and use information technology. They must recognize the role of the doctor in society and their place in the hospital or community care team. They must be able to make sensible career decisions and sell themselves successfully, so that they can get the specialist jobs that they want. Once consultants, their clinical expertise will be an important part of the team-based care of patients, but they must also be able to manage, organize and educate other members of the team. Later, as clinical directors, or in private practice, doctors must develop a business-like approach to managing money, negotiating and working with other people. Throughout their career, doctors must know how to delegate and when to seek help. The skills discussed in this book are required by everyone who cares for patients, so they have been termed 'generic skills' or 'over-arching competencies'.

Many books aimed at businessmen discuss aspects of personal skill development, but their advice usually has limited relevance to doctors. For several years, the authors of this book have tutored medical trainees to prepare them for job interviews and consultancy. This book originated from these *ad hoc* tutorials. We hope that it will be a practical source of information which will help doctors become effective consultants.

The information in this book is accurate at the time of writing, but health care is changing rapidly and this may result in changes that we cannot anticipate.

Many colleagues have contributed to this book by commenting on what we have written. We would welcome suggestions on how it might be improved in future.

Chris Johnson
Colin Hall
Frances Forrest

ABOUT THE AUTHORS

Dr Chris Johnson MA MD FRCA
Chris Johnson worked for his research degree in environmental physiology while overwintering at Halley base in Antarctica. On returning to the UK, he trained in anaesthetics and is now a consultant in Bristol. He has been a college tutor in anaesthetics and chairman of a hospital medical audit committee. He is particularly interested in improving methods of teaching practical skills, and in techniques of assessment.

Dr Colin Hall MB BS FRCA
Colin Hall is an intensivist in Bristol, UK. As a post-graduate tutor for several years he established assessment systems for junior trainees, sought to improve the quality of training in many specialties and chaired a regional tutors' committee. He is interested in the ethics of modern health care.

Dr Frances Forrest MB BS FRCA
Frances Forrest trained in Bristol, UK, and the USA and spent a period working with 'Project Orbis' — a flying eye hospital which seeks to raise the standards of ophthalmic care throughout the world by educating local health workers. She has diploma in health management and is currently involved in setting up the anaesthetic and surgical simulator in Bristol.

Acknowledgements

The book contains material from many sources. Over the years, when we have attended a particularly good talk or read a useful article, we have jotted down ideas for our own use. Later, we cannot always remember where they came from. So, if you recognize any of your ideas in what we have written, thank you — imitation is the sincerest form of flattery.

Dr Paul Upton originally encouraged us to write this book and introduced us to the team at BIOS. Our trainees and colleagues at Southmead and the Bristol Royal Infirmary suggested many of the topics that we have included and many of them have criticized what we have written. We thank them all for their contributions.

Dr Neville Goodman expertly suggested numerous ways to improve our writing.

1. GETTING A JOB

Objectives of this section

- to enable you to make sensible career choices
- to explain the stages of the appointments process
- to enable you to write an effective application form and curriculum vitae (CV)
- to prepare you for a job interview

Getting good jobs is crucial to your career. The jobs you obtain affect the experience you gain, and so alter your chances of being appointed to a desirable consultant post. Time and effort are needed if you are to succeed (Box 1.1).

Box 1.1. Stages in the appointments procedure

- Career planning
- Preparation
- Producing a CV
- Selecting a referee
- The advertisement
- Job descriptions

- Short-listing
- Visits
- Interview
- Success or rejection
- Induction procedures

Because they must comply with equal opportunities legislation, health organizations are introducing 'structured' appointment procedures in which the 'person specification', candidate logbook, and structured references are replacing the CV and letter of reference. Sadly, each organization is developing its own regulations, and variations occur. The instructions in this chapter should enable you to avoid common pitfalls which prevent you being short-listed.

Career planning

Before looking for a job, consider your priorities and rank them. Your list might include the factors in Box 1.2.

The order in which you rank these factors is likely to change as you progress up the career ladder. This exercise should enable you to select a few posts for further consideration. Everyone needs help and advice when they apply for a job. During the most important stage of your training, that is during your registrar years, you should aim to obtain a job in a centre of excellence as this will then enable you to become a competitive applicant for desirable

---

Box 1.2. Factors influencing job choice

- The type of clinical work you want to do
- The training you will receive
- Opportunities for performing research
- The colleagues with whom you will work
- The number of trainees that you will work with or teach
- Conditions of employment and hours of work
- On-call commitments
- Salary and amount of private practice available
- The area where you would like to live
- Ease of travel to major urban centres
- Family preferences

---

consultant posts. The location of your training centre may affect where you spend the rest of your life, as trainees more often obtain consultant posts near to their training city.

Although there is greater job mobility than there used to be, a consultant post is still regarded as a long-term commitment. It is essential to try to find a senior post which you can enjoy. A nice hospital, pleasant colleagues, skilled staff and good management contribute to making work worthwhile.

You must assess the competition in your specialty. If you possess unusual sought-after skills, you can be very selective; but if you are in a competitive specialty with many equivalently qualified doctors seeking jobs, you must be prepared to compromise and apply for any decent job that is advertised, not simply ones that are convenient geographically. Usually it is reasonable to wait a few weeks for the job you want to be advertised, but if the delay will be longer you should consider your second choices. If you have failed to be appointed to a particular post, you are probably unwise to wait until that job is re-advertised, however encouraging the department appeared after your initial interview.

Preparation

Once you have decided, explore your chances of getting the job you would like. Contact the chairman of your chosen department, or the training co-ordinator of the registrar scheme. Find out: how the department or scheme is organized, how keen staff are to teach, what research is going on, and the usual standard of job applicants. In particular, discover whether certain criteria are used during the short-listing process — for instance that you must have attended certain courses, or passed certain examinations. Competition for a popular job means that the qualifications for a candidate to be short-listed can be much higher than the essential requirements stated in the person specification. You may be able to find out when a post will be advertised. Try to obtain enough information to decide whether to wait for your chosen job to be advertised, or whether it would be wiser to apply elsewhere. If the people you visit appear evasive, don't blame them; the jobs market fluctuates and they have to be cautious in what they say.

Before visiting a department or applying for a job, you should ensure that your CV is accurate and up-to-date.

Producing a curriculum vitae   SKILL LEVEL 1

In the medical world, your CV is your passport to success. It must be an accurate statement of what you have done in your career, and must be attractively presented so that you sell yourself to future employers. A typical CV will include:

1. Title page
Your full name and qualifications
The title of the job you are applying for

2. Personal details
Name
Date of birth and age
Home address and work address
Contact telephone/fax/e-mail numbers
Marital status and children (commonly included, but not required)
Education
Secondary education and higher examinations
University and medical school
Prizes and awards
Degrees and diploma (dates and awarding bodies)
Accreditation date
GMC registration number
Medical insurance/protection society number
Overseas candidates must state clearly that they have appropriate permit-free training time to enable them to complete the advertised job.
Note that, as a result of their equal opportunities policy, certain employers request that some of this information is excluded from your application. Read the instructions.

3. Medical posts held
There is debate about the best way to list these. Chronological order is the easiest for an assessor to understand. If there are gaps in your career, these should be explained in the next section, otherwise the employer may assume the worst: jail, nervous breakdown or extended holiday.

4. Description of experience gained
This should be succinct, but informative. Details of rotas or saying a job is 'busy' are valueless but descriptions of the skills you gained during a job can

be useful. All experience is valuable. If you have done something unusual, for instance been an expedition doctor or an athlete on a sporting tour, explain it. Maternity leave should be noted, but does not require further explanation. This section of your CV may eventually be relegated to your personal profile/portfolio (see p. 6) if this concept becomes popular.

5. Research
A comprehensive list of your publications with full details of all authors. Use a standard method of citing the publications, such as the Vancouver convention, and ensure that the references are given accurately. A summary of the results of your research and your role in the project is desirable. You should make it clear whether papers were research articles published in a peer-reviewed journal or simply letters, abstracts or articles accepted by an editor.

6. Audit
Most trainees should have participated in medical or clinical audit studies during the course of their training. Summarize your involvement and the findings.

7. Presentations
Lectures or presentations to departments or learned societies.

8. Membership of professional societies

9. Professional responsibilities
Membership of committees and posts held on them.

10. Acquisition of 'personal' skills
Though not yet universal, it is becoming increasingly important to list the personal skills you have acquired in management, education, training and organization. If you speak any foreign languages or are competent at using computer databases, spreadsheets or word-processing packages, these skills should be listed.

11. Postgraduate courses attended
Many applicants now provide a list of the courses they have attended. Some specialities require that trainees attend an Advanced Life Support course or specialist skills courses. If attendance at such courses is mandatory, they may be included in the personal details section.

12. Hobbies and interests
This section always interests the interview panel and they will question you on it. You should have a specific expertise in an area before claiming it as an interest. For instance an interest in photography would suggest that you should either collect cameras, develop your own pictures for exhibition or

be good enough to exhibit prints and get some published. An interest in travel implies something more than going overseas on a package tour once a year. Few doctors can manage to play more than two sports well and still perform their clinical duties. However, definitely mention any team that you have represented at university, county or national level. Several well-known surgeons have represented their country at rugby. Include musical skills and qualifications in this section.

13. Statement of intent
Many CVs now include a brief statement of the candidate's intentions, and why they have selected the advertised post.

14. List your referees
If these are not stated elsewhere in the application. Your referee will not be impressed if you spell his or her name incorrectly or use the wrong initials. If you are unsure, ask, or go to the library and look up the name in the medical register.

Important points about CVs
General presentation
Your CV must be neat, accurate, spelt correctly, and printed cleanly. For consultant applications it is essential that the date you will receive your certificate of completion of specialist training (CCST) has been confirmed by your college. False claims made on CVs or job application forms can lead to dismissal and legal proceedings.

Brevity is desirable. A list of procedures performed under supervision, and by yourself, is more impressive than waffle about the stress of a job or the size of a unit. Always get the draft checked by an experienced assessor. Expect to write at least four drafts to get the CV right. The exact layout does not matter, choose one that suits your style and looks tidy. Only produce the CV yourself if you are competent at word-processing; if you are a poor typist persuade the departmental secretary to produce it, or use a professional agency. Having produced your CV, proof-read it very carefully, photocopy it onto good quality paper, check the page order, and staple it together in the correct order. Special binders are usually unnecessary and just get added to the employer's stocks before the CV is read.

Tailoring the CV
Your CV should match the job advertised. Assessors expect that the title page will state the job that you are applying for, and the text should emphasize your abilities in the fields that the job requires. When employers have produced a person specification (see p. 8), you must tailor your CV to emphasize the essential and desirable characteristics that they seek.

Selection of referees

Select your referees with care. Discuss your application with your chosen doctor and ask if they will act for you. Cautious responses should be noted and an alternative offered 'if you are too busy'. It is foolish to rely on a referee who feels able to offer only half-hearted support. Do not supply doctors names as referees if you have not discussed your job application with them. Supply your referees with an up-to-date copy of your CV and keep them informed about the progress of your applications. Diligent referees may vary their reference according to the job that you are applying for, but are unlikely to be able to do so if unexpected requests arrive at short notice. For senior posts, referees will usually be either nationally known figures, the college tutor or department chairman. Other referees are suitable either if you have had close clinical contacts with them or if they have supervised a research or audit project.

Problems with CVs

The most common problem is that people hide their talents. Employers will not read between the lines to discover your true worth. List all your skills succinctly and clearly. It is difficult to select the best from a group of very similar CVs and any excuse will be taken to exclude you from further consideration. Badly presented, inaccurate, scruffy or misspelt CVs demonstrate that you are either a careless individual or have put little effort into your job application. Dot matrix printing and handwritten corrections to CVs create a bad impression. Such faults mean that you will not be short-listed.

Personal profiles

Although still uncommon in the medical profession, 'personal profiles' form part of career development and appointments procedures in other professions. The 'profile' is a file which includes documentation of your acquisition of skills. It would include your university degree certificates and post-graduate diplomas, summaries of your case logbook, and attendance certificates for courses. Other relevant information such as your GMC annual registration certificate, protection society certificate and records of vaccination should be included. Many people feel that 'personal profiles' are just another example of irritating bureaucracy, but routinely storing this information together can save you time when you have to complete application forms.

The job application

Most British medical jobs are advertised in the *British Medical Journal* (*BMJ*) supplement and on the *BMJ* Internet Website (www.bmj.com). They may also be advertised in journals such as *Hospital Doctor*. The job you want may be advertised only once and the whole appointments procedure brief. Look at the advertisements each week, and if you go on holiday, make sure someone watches the journals for you. Late applications are usually rejected.

The advertisement and job information pack

Most advertisements say little. If you are interested in a job, apply for the job information pack. Until recently, these have also contained limited information, although they are improving. They should consist of an application form, the person specification and the job description; additionally many Trusts now provide a propaganda leaflet containing more information about the organization and nearby facilities.

Job descriptions are often very comprehensive, but may not tell you what you want to know. Read them carefully and see what they say, not only about the job, but also about accommodation, removal expenses, library facilities, study leave and so forth. Trainees should find out who will be their educational supervisor, and what courses are available nearby. Hours of work should be defined; nowadays this is as important for consultant appointments, where there are no limits on hours of work, as it is for trainee posts where there are national controls.

Until recently the clinical skills and interests of a candidate for a consultant appointment were taken for granted, but nowadays job descriptions are designed to enable a trust to achieve its business aims. After appointment, consultants used to be able to develop their own clinical and research interests; now, if a trust has a contract to fulfil in, for instance, hip replacement surgery, it is likely to demand that the appointed clinician spends most of their theatre time working in this sub-specialty.

Trusts and training rotations are producing more comprehensive *person specifications* in which the essential and desirable characteristics of the doctor they seek are listed. An example of a person specification for a registrar post is given in Box 1.3.

For senior posts, the person specification may indicate the needs of the Trust. Are they trying to attract an experienced doctor who is looking for a long-term post, or a person who is developing their skills and might want to stay for a shorter time to gain experience? What clinical and non-clinical skills are thought important?

The *trust information package*, if it exists, usually contains a few pictures of local beauty spots, a smiling patient and a picture of the Trust's least ugly building! This may be unhelpful but, like an estate agent's brochure, you may be able to form an impression of what the Trust's priorities are. If you are lucky, it will tell you about accommodation, when you can get a hot meal and how much you will pay to park cars. It is up to you to discover the strengths and weaknesses of the hospital you are applying to.

Box 1.3. Person specification for specialist registrar post

	Essential criteria	Desirable criteria
Qualifications	MB BS or equivalent primary college examination	Other relevant qualifications ALS/ACLS/ATLS or equivalent
Experience	Two years in specialty Attendance at basic skills course Evidence of smooth progression through training programmes Logbook of experience	Six months to one year as a senior house officer (SHO) in other relevant fields
Ability and knowledge	Capable of managing basic clinical problems safely and effectively without supervision	Neat, legible completion of notes and charts Computer skills
Clinical and technical skills	Appropriate to specialty	Appropriate to specialty
Audit	Understands principles of audit	Completion of criterion-based audit
Research		Understands research principles
Motivation	Commitment to specialty Commitment to self-learning Punctual Reliable	Initiative
Personality	Good at crisis management Able to cope with stress Good communication skills Fluent English speaker Conscientious Honest	Ability to lead Works well in teams Patience Sense of humour Presentation skills
Management		Ability to organize
Other requirements	Willing to work in locations as specified in job description General Medical Council (GMC) registration Hepatitis B immune Willing to enter into training agreement with post-graduate dean	Current driving licence

Initial contacts

The information package should contain contact telephone numbers. Many large hospitals and rotations discourage SHO and registrar applicants from visiting between a job advertisement and short-listing. This is a matter of practicality: having large numbers of candidates visiting a hospital is a waste of time and might unfairly penalize candidates from far away. Smaller organizations may want to see all candidates at this stage. Most trusts encourage potential consultant applicants to visit to discover more about the job before they submit their application. It is sensible to telephone the relevant department, explain that you may apply for the job, and ask if they would like to see you before short-listing.

Completing the job application

If you decide to apply for the job you will need to complete the necessary application forms. Each section must be answered comprehensively and tidily; responding with 'see CV' is not acceptable, and may count against you. Separate sheets should be attached to the application form if its boxes are too small. Take as much care with this form as you did with your CV and ensure that you compare your skills with the mandatory and desirable attributes listed in the person specification. Return the application form to the staffing office together with the correct number of copies of your CV and, traditionally, a neatly handwritten letter explaining which job you are applying for. All these documents will be used for selecting the candidates to be short-listed.

Employers need to see a number of documents before you take up your job. These include:

- GMC registration certificate
- Notification of immunization status against Hepatitis B
- Occupational health forms
- Declaration form concerning previous criminal convictions

You may be asked to include copies of relevant documents with your application form.

The appointments procedure

Short-listing

Short-listing is undertaken solely on the basis of the job application form and the CV. Candidates are assessed against the job specification, usually under a number of headings such as:

- Pre-medical qualifications
- Medical qualifications
- Post-graduate courses attended
- Present and previous jobs and skills acquired

- Research experience and writing
- Educational skills and teaching experience
- Administrative and managerial skills
- Interests outside medicine

These headings may be further sub-divided according to the essential and desirable attributes listed in the person specification. Under equal opportunities legislation, racial origin, gender and marital status must play no part in the selection process, and candidates who feel that they have been unjustly excluded can take the case to an industrial tribunal. Many businesses exclude candidates over a particular age; in medicine this is unusual as many doctors have followed complex career pathways which have increased their skills and experience.

Short-listed candidates will be invited to interview and told if they will be expected to make a presentation to the appointments committee.

The pre-interview visit

The pre-interview visit is an important opportunity for you to gain an impression of the department and find out details of the job. It will also be a chance for members of that department to learn about you. Regardless of your personal views about the importance of dress, you would be wise to make sure that you are wearing tidy clothes, have clean shoes and are respectably turned out. Suits resurrected from the sixth-form at school and scuffed shoes do not create the appearance of someone keen to get a job. You should have prepared a list of questions to ask — topics that were not covered in detail in the job description, and you should be prepared to answer anything thrown at you. Take care answering these questions: be natural, but be aware that a glib throwaway remark may affect people's view of you.

For senior job appointments, you may need to make several visits, and you may find that your welcome varies at each visit. You should make considerable efforts to see all the senior staff in your chosen department as failure to make contact may count against you. Before short-listing, you will probably find that the department is very friendly and inviting. Existing consultants will be keen to make you interested in applying for their job and want to sell themselves so that they get a good list of applicants. After short-listing their attitude may appear to alter, with the questioning becoming more aggressive and intense. This is not a personal threat to you. Do not be surprised; it is because they are keen to find out about you and whether you will suit their requirements. Make sure that you visit all key figures, not forgetting to offer to visit the Trust Chief Executive and Medical Director. You will also need to get a feel for how much the trust wants your skills. It is becoming more common for consultants in shortage specialties to be offered incentives to choose a specific trust, either in the form of additional salary increments or favourable removal expenses.

Preparation for the interview

You cannot predict what you will be asked, but it will be assumed that you have done your homework. Before a consultant interview decide what your plans are if you obtain the post, and what you can offer to the trust. You should read relevant documents produced by the National Health Service (NHS) executive, royal colleges, professional associations and confidential enquiries. You should also find out whether the Trust has produced any strategic or business plans that might affect your work, and have some understanding of the views of the stakeholders in the hospital (GPs, purchasers, patient groups, etc.).

As a trainee you will be expected to know about relevant medico-political controversies and have informed views on research, audit, education and training. Try to organize at least one mock interview before the real thing; listen carefully to the comments made by experienced interviewers.

Presentations

Some appointments committees now ask the candidate make a presentation. The value of this is disputed, but subjects have included:
'How will this job improve your career?'
'How will your appointment improve health care in our local community?'
'The value of your research'
'How could our organization better meet the targets in the Patient's Charter?'
'What will be the role of the District General Hospital in 20 years time?'
Candidates need to be quite clear about what is required of them and whether they will be allowed or expected to use visual aids.

The interview

The composition of interview committees for most posts is governed by statute. You ought to be informed who will sit on the committee before you attend, and a bit of background research into their clinical interests can pay dividends. Most medical interviews are structured, with similar questions being asked of each candidate. If you are interviewed early, maintain a discrete silence about what you were asked. You should assume that all candidates enter the interview room with an equal chance of obtaining the job, so be confident. This may, or may not, be true, but a tentative performance can lose you a job that you were favoured for.

Typically an interview begins with a number of easy and non-aggressive questions to allow the candidate to settle into their chair and adjust to the interview panel. More detailed questioning follows. Although interview training is improving matters, not all interviewers are equally good. You should be asked a series of 'open' questions. A question is said to be *closed* if the answer is likely to be predictable and *open* if the answer is not in part defined by the question, Open questions will yield more information, many closed questions can be answered by a simple 'yes' or 'no'. For example if the professor asks 'Do you enjoy research?', the inevitable reply to such a closed question is likely to be 'yes' (unless the candidate is an honest fool). If the professor asks a more open question such as 'Why should a doctor do research?' the response is likely to be a set of positive reasons. The true feelings of the candidate will only be discovered by asking the truly open question 'What do you think are the advantages and drawbacks of spending some time doing medical research?'.

Whatever you are asked, think carefully, answer the question that was asked — not something completely different, look at your questioner, and speak up. Jobs often go to people with a gleam in their eye and obvious enthusiasm, even if they do not have the best CV. Most candidates would do twice as well by saying half-as-much. If you do not understand something, ask the questioner to rephrase. The chairperson of the committee should protect you from intrusive personal questions; if you feel that a question is inappropriate, you should politely refuse to answer it. Persistent questioning that has racial or sexual overtones should be reported to the appointing authority giving details of the questions asked and your responses.

Questioning will usually proceed around the table, with the main topics of discussion being:

- Past achievements from your CV
- Skills and expertise
- Future plans
- Research
- Management experience and skills
- Audit, training and education
- Personal attributes

At the end the chairperson should ask if you have any questions of the interview panel. The best answer is to say 'no' — you really should have discovered everything about the job long before you get to this stage in the process. When a structured interview system is being used, the interviewers may be expected to score or grade each of your answers. It may be disconcerting to see them making notes as you talk, but they have to justify why they appointed or rejected you and provide appropriate documentation to the medical staffing department.

Discussion

Once all the candidates have been interviewed, the panel must make their choice. Sometimes the winner is obvious and the task easy. At other times it is difficult, especially if similar candidates have attracted powerful support from different camps. Particularly at consultant level, many factors influence who is appointed and the successful candidate is not necessarily the one with the best paper qualifications. At all stages in your career there is an element of luck. All you can do is keep your fingers crossed!

Afterwards

Once the decision has been made, and any legal or health reports considered, the successful candidate is offered the post. Unsuccessful candidates ought to get feedback on why they did not get the job, but this can be a difficult task for a member of the committee who is faced with a despairing candidate, and it is not always done effectively.

Success or rejection

Success is great, but now you must negotiate a starting date suitable for both your new and old employers. All medical jobs now begin on the first Wednesday of the month. Try to make sure that you will have an induction course before starting your clinical duties. Find out from the personnel officer how to claim expenses for your visits and your move.

Not everyone can be lucky. Failure to get appointed at an interview is disappointing but does not necessarily mean that you are less good than the appointed candidates, it may be simply that you performed less well on the day. You should get debriefed by a member of the panel who may be able to tell you your strengths and weaknesses. Make sure that you tell your referees of your success or failure.

Induction procedures

Over the years, doctors moving to a new job have been expected to fend for themselves. This unsatisfactory state of affairs may still apply for senior posts, but usually trainee medical staff now have to attend an induction course.

A good employer will have produced a 'welcoming package'. At the very least, a new arrival should be given the information listed in Box 1.4.

If the hospital you join cannot provide this information for you, you could usefully set about producing a package for your successor.

Box 1.4. Arrival requirements for new doctors

- Be provided with appropriate identity badges
- Know where to park their car and be provided with appropriate passes
- Know how to get into the department out of hours
- Have access to secure storage for personal effects
- Have a method of communication (telephone/pager/mobile phone/computer)
- Have office space and a desk
- Know where to get secretarial assistance
- Have immediate access to the local IT system, including training, and access to the local patient care systems and e-mail
- Have access to library and post-graduate centre
- Know where information is kept about clinical protocols and hospital policies such as the major incident plan, coroners' referrals, security, fire procedures and manual handling policies
- Know where to eat, and where to find a bedroom if resident on-call.
- Have a guided tour of relevant clinical areas and be introduced to key clinical and support staff
- Be informed of the local management structure and be introduced to relevant people
- Know about local sport and leisure facilities

Related topics

Advice (p. 20)
Writing a reference (p. 137)

2. ORGANIZING YOURSELF

Objectives of this section

- to enable you to work efficiently
- to demonstrate how you can control your workload
- to help you minimize personal stress
- to illustrate the benefits of being assertive
- to suggest where you should seek advice

Some people fit more into life than others. Effective personal organization reduces stress and increases efficiency. Some doctors are naturally efficient, others learn to work efficiently, while the rest remain disorganized throughout their lives — to the despair of patients, colleagues and secretaries.

Time management

When you begin work as a house officer your schedule may seem to be governed by factors outside your own control. Despite this, some junior doctors achieve more than others. Box 2.1 lists simple concepts of time management. The most important of these principles is to plan your work efficiently.

Box 2.1. Basic principles for organizing work

- A little planning early in the day saves time and frustration later
- Tackle important tasks when fresh
- Work expands to fill the time available: allocate specific lengths of time to particular tasks and try not to exceed them
- Overwork and stress reduce efficiency. Allocate time for eating and relaxation
- Avoid postponing unpleasant or boring tasks; they won't improve with keeping
- Perfection and efficiency may sometimes be incompatible; efficiency is often, but not always, the better goal
- Twenty per cent of people's time achieves 80% of their total productivity

---

Keeping track of work

The simplest way to organize your work is to keep an accurate and up-to-date diary, Filofax or electronic organizer. Filofaxes and electronic organizers allow more information to be stored in one place than diaries and mean that you do not have to transcribe information at the start of each year.

Two diaries are not better than one, and can mislead if information is not correlated regularly. If you have a secretary, be clear who has the master diary. Your list of appointments should always be available so that possible clashes can be spotted at the time that meetings are booked. Entries should be unambiguous, giving dates, times, and locations of meetings and the reasons for them. Get into the habit of reviewing your diary at the start of each week and the beginning of each day so that you can plan your schedule.

Routine

A set routine, known to colleagues, increases efficiency. If you are in your office at a particular time each day, people can save up their telephone calls rather than trying to contact you throughout the day. A group of house officers who arranges a ward round at a regular time each evening is less likely to be disturbed than one without a routine.

When you become a consultant, it will help people in your team if they know when you welcome being contacted and when you do not. A period in the weekly schedule when you have an 'open door' policy means that you can concentrate unexpected diversions. Equally important, clinical emergencies apart, it is helpful if periods can be built into the week when you can get on with tasks uninterrupted by colleagues, telephone or bleep.

Making contact

Instant communication is the curse of doctors' lives. A phone call or bleep is a strident demand for attention, regardless of priority. Message pagers are better than bleeps because you can assess what priority to give to the response. Senior staff can overcome the problem of unwanted telephone calls by using their secretaries as a filter; junior medical staff have no such protection. If you know someone is busy, only telephone or bleep them if you have to; save up less vital messages for a quiet time of day, or send them a letter, fax or e-mail.

Lists

Two minutes' organization early in a day can save a lot of time later. Write down what you need to do. The skill comes in arranging these tasks efficiently.

Work consists of *fixed* and *flexible* tasks. Fixed tasks are those that must be done at a particular time, such as ward rounds, operating lists, out-patient clinics or formal meetings. Other jobs can be organized flexibly around these commitments, but bear in mind that certain goals must be achieved by particular times of day. For example, before a ward round a house officer must: review patients, obtain the results of their recent investigations and ensure that their clinical notes are up-to-date.

One way to organize daily work is by *priority* and to give preference to simple tasks that can be completed quickly. This apparently simple method is recommended in many management books and is effective for office staff, but is often inefficient if you work in a big hospital. The problem is that boring, dull or lengthy tasks get shunted down the list and are tackled only when failure to do so will cause a crisis. Furthermore, you may end up making many unnecessary journeys around the hospital. It is usually more efficient for a doctor to group tasks by time or place.

Grouping jobs by *time* means that you must think ahead. For example, dictation is best done early in the day, so that your secretary can have the correspondence available for you to sign before you go home. Outgoing telephone calls can be made at the same time as you deal with the morning mail. Less time is wasted if there is a delay contacting someone, and if they are not available you can send an e-mail or arrange with their secretary to phone back. As a more junior doctor, review your patients early in the day and list their needs. One spell at the computer will then enable you to review the previous day's results and order appropriate additional investigations and drugs. While completing this task ensure that you prescribe discharge drugs for patients leaving the hospital. Accurate and timely paperwork reduces the number of calls you get from nurses or pharmacists. Ideally, these tasks should be completed before the nurses need you to admit new patients.

Geographical organization can also save time. If you have several jobs to do in distant parts of the hospital, combine them so that you only make a single trip around the site. Decide the most effective way to perform each task: a personal visit, an e-mail, or a telephone call. Delegate jobs where appropriate, but only if this will increase everyone's efficiency.

Emergencies
In medicine unexpected problems are common and it is wise to build time into your routine to allow for the unexpected. It is rarely possible to complete an anticipated 4 hours work within a half-day slot, so it is better to plan to achieve a bit less.

Critical path analysis
Advance planning may prevent crises. In the simplest terms, if you are absent minded, a diary note saying 'Daughter's birthday next week' prompts you to buy a card before it is too late. Critical path analysis is a method of organizing a complex project so that significant deadlines are recognized well in advance and plans made to ensure that a routine matter does not become a crisis because it has been overlooked. If you are invited to give a lecture, you need to have the script written well in advance, audio-visual (A-V) aids designed and sent to the medical illustration department, and study leave booked several weeks before the day of the lecture. Noting the

medical illustrations department deadline in your diary ensures that you don't have to plead to have your art work fast-tracked. Many people only perform well when they are put under pressure. The introduction of a series of deadlines in the critical path analysis focuses attention on the progress of a complex project and ensures that the overall task is completed smoothly.

Sadly, many NHS managers seem to work on the 'fire fighting' or crisis management principle, which inevitably annoys doctors asked to deal urgently with last-minute paperwork.

Information technology

Computers are altering the way some doctors work radically. Computerized clinical and pathological databases make it easier to obtain information about patients, even if their paper records are missing. Messages can be sent by e-mail without having to locate the recipient. Some hospital information systems allow doctors at home to link into their e-mail, pathology and imaging systems, so enabling clinical decisions to be made effectively from a distance. Learning to use these systems may be a worthwhile investment of time, but beware of enthusiasts for the technology; computers are helpful only if they save you time.

Assertion

Being assertive is not the same as being aggressive. Assertion is making clear your views on an issue and, in the context of work, making other people understand that you do or do not want to undertake a task. You will upset fewer people if you decline a task firmly but politely than if you accept it with a vague phrase like 'I'll see what I can do' and then do nothing. Clearly, the way you seek or refuse a task makes a difference to people's impression of you. At times in your career you will be expected to contribute to a department or organization by taking on jobs that you would prefer not to do, and then you should try to do them well. It is more efficient to gather a portfolio of related tasks than it is to achieve a little in several unrelated fields. Do not take on more than you can handle; you will simply upset everyone by under-performing on all your jobs.

Assertion is also about dealing on an equal footing with colleagues. Some people will always seek to dominate others, ignoring their needs and aspirations. It is sensible and acceptable to make it clear that, while respecting the rights of others, you too have a point of view that deserves an equal hearing. Non-assertive individuals become the passive pawns of dominant personalities and become stressed because work patterns are manipulated to their disadvantage and the credit for their achievements is claimed by others. Often they are unable to express themselves and are ignored by others, leading to problems with self-esteem. They may be sensitive to criticism and may bottle up feelings, all of which add to the stress.

The personal characteristics listed in Box 2.2 should not cause you stress. Developing confidence in dealing with these situations will be associated with the development of appropriate body language including better eye contact. Many organizations now run assertiveness training courses which are valuable to people who find it difficult to express their views.

Box 2.2. Characteristics of being appropriately assertive

- Clarifying your own ideas of what you think and want
- Being prepared to express your own opinions clearly and to argue for them
- Being prepared to offer solutions to problems, not just moaning
- Initiating conversations
- Being prepared to offer advice and information
- Making sure that you get someone to clarify a point if you have not understood
- Being happy to request services or information
- Being prepared to confront someone who is behaving wrongly or inappropriately

---

Stress

Some stress is desirable if you are to perform well. Boredom leads to poor performance of routine duties. Most people perform best at interviews or as lecturers if they are stressed by the prospect. However, excessive stress, particularly when caused by many different factors, reduces performance. Ultimately there may be the complete withdrawal from normal activities that is known as a 'nervous breakdown' (Box 2.3).

Box 2.3. Serious stresses

- Poor interpersonal relationships at home or work
- Changes in status: marriage, childbirth, bereavement
- Personal or family illness
- Change in work: promotion, relocation or unemployment
- Moving house
- Financial worries
- Serious problems at work, including a negligence claim or a clinical disaster
- Racial or sexual harassment
- Examinations

Hard work by itself is only stressful if it gets out of control. Always allow an appropriate amount of time for socializing, recreation and for your family. You are probably becoming excessively overloaded if your working day regularly overruns, your family feel neglected or you cannot enjoy your normal recreational activities because of work commitments. Excessive alcohol consumption, fatigue, headaches or persistent indigestion are serious physical warning signs of problems.

Stress reduction

Simple techniques can reduce stress. Organize yourself, control your workload and limit the demands other people make of you, so that you have time for what you want to do. This requires appropriate assertion and you may have to be taught these skills if you are having problems. You may find some situations such as interviews or viva examinations particularly frightening, and under-perform as a result. Relaxation therapy can reduce stress; meditation and breathing and relaxation exercises help. Hospital clinical psychologists will usually know someone who specializes in teaching these skills.

Doctors frequently look after each other poorly. If you sense that one of your colleagues is particularly stressed, it is worth trying to talk to them or to draw the attention of a more senior member of staff to their plight. People under the greatest stress rarely admit their problems, and may need someone else to confront them. Failure to do so can lead to dramatic consequences such as a suicide attempt. Sadly, people who successfully commit suicide rarely give any external indications of the stress that they have bottled up, but they frequently leave behind them considerable feelings of guilt and helplessness among their colleagues, who wonder if they could have helped more.

Advice

Everyone needs help and advice at some time. There are many ways that doctors can obtain both professional and personal help.

Professional advice

You should get advice from several sources before choosing a specialty or applying for a job.

Consultants are usually willing to suggest how trainees can develop their careers. As a junior thinking about a specialist career, seek advice both from senior members of your present firm and from senior staff in other specialties.

College tutors are appointed by Royal Colleges to supervise training in a particular specialty at the hospital level. Career registrars requiring professional advice should seek advice from them. They can advise juniors thinking of a career in their specialty about the qualifications and skills they will need.

Training co-ordinators/programme directors are consultants who run rotational training programmes for a specialty. They have a good idea of when jobs will become available and the sort of attributes that candidates need to be short-listed. You should contact this consultant before applying for a job on the scheme he or she organizes.

Post-graduate clinical tutors are responsible for supervizing the training of pre-registration house officers (PRHOs) and SHOs who have not yet joined a specialty training rotation. A junior doctor should seek their advice if they have a professional or personal problem.

Regional educational advisors are Royal College appointees responsible for professional specialty standards in a region. They are a useful source of advice for senior trainees as they have a broad view of professional standards in their specialty.

Post-graduate dean's office. Post-graduate deans have overall responsibility for supervising trainees. They organize regular reviews of progress. Advice can be sought at these reviews. Candidates with difficulties can discuss their problems at separate interviews. This mechanism is most suited to the senior trainee who is finding serious career problems.

Royal Colleges, faculties and associations supply general information pamphlets which can help medical students and junior doctors to decide on their career. Some colleges have professional advisers whose task is to assist doctors who are finding it difficult to pass examinations.

Personal help

Poor interpersonal relationships, exhaustion, financial troubles and professional conflicts all produce personal stress and impede professional performance. Many doctors are reluctant to seek help, but there are times in life when having someone to talk to can help.

Friends and colleagues should be a source of assistance. People are often reluctant to seek help, but many people will willingly give aid when asked.

Post-graduate clinical tutors can often help trainees who feel that they cannot get on with their professional colleagues and are particularly suited to dealing with situations where there is felt to be personal antagonism, or sexual or racial harassment.

Clinical psychologists in some hospitals provide stress counselling.

The *British Medical Association* runs a confidential counselling telephone line for doctors under stress. The telephone number is 0645 200169.

Chaplains visit all hospitals and can provide staff with solace particularly at times of great emotional stress. Hospital chaplains deal with all sorts of people and lack of formal religious conviction should not prevent you from seeking help from these skilled communicators.

Health

General practitioners. All doctors should register with a GP and make use of their services. Doctors are prone to consulting their colleagues or self-medication and this is usually not a good idea.

Occupational health departments advise about matters in which health affects a person's ability to perform their job. The occupational health consultant must be informed if a doctor is unable to perform clinical duties properly because of ill health (for instance back injury) or has become a hazard to patients (seroconversion or alcoholism). The department may be able to offer counselling and treatment. Bear in mind that the department may have to pass information about the employee to the employing authority.

Sick doctors' schemes. Both within hospitals and within some professional groups, there are confidential mechanisms such as *The Three Wise Men* which exist to support and counsel doctors who are felt to be seriously under-performing as a result of health or other problems. Senior medical staff will know how to activate these systems. All clinicians have a duty to ensure that appropriate help is given to colleagues whose physical or psychological health has deteriorated such that patients might be harmed.

The *General Medical Council* has always been responsible for regulating doctors' professional standards, but until recently was unable to deal with matters of clinical competence. The GMC is now developing procedures designed to ensure that incompetent doctors can be assessed, and either helped to improve or removed from the medical register (see p. 162).

Contracts

Doctors are often naïve at dealing with finance and contracts. Early advice can save grief later.

British Medical Association. The professional officers of the British Medical Association offer advice about medical contracts and professional standards. Consult them before any non-standard employment contract is signed. They also provide information about remuneration for extra-contractual work and removal expenses, which is particularly important when taking up a consultant post or accepting a partnership agreement. Hospitals will usually have a place of work accredited representative (POWAR), who is a doctor who represents doctors professional interests at trade union negotiations on pay and terms of service.

Professional associations. The royal colleges are charitable educational foundations. They are barred from offering advice on employment matters. Some specialties have professional associations to offer information on what constitutes a reasonable workload and what facilities are required by a doctor in a particular specialty.

Defence unions/protection societies. The medical defence companies are highly skilled at assisting doctors who have a serious clinical problem or who are accused of professional negligence or incompetence. Every doctor should belong to one, as Trust medical indemnity is designed to protect the organization, not the individual doctor. Defence unions will assist with professional complaints against a doctor, but will not deal with employment matters.

Accountancy. Doctors should ensure that their personal finances, private practice accounts and charitable donations for research or departments do not become entangled. Professional advice should be sought from bank managers, independent accountants and employing authorities.

Related topics

Career planning (p. 1)
Counselling (p. 33)
Mentoring (p. 34)

3. STRUCTURED TRAINING

Objectives of this section
- to understand why 'structured training' has been introduced
- to explain the principles of assessment, counselling and mentoring
- to enable you to use an assessment meeting effectively

Structure of medical education in the UK

Until the Calman reforms of 1996 most British medical training was based upon an apprenticeship within a consultant 'firm'. Trainees spent 10–15 years as a 'junior' before obtaining their consultant post, which typically became a job for life. A high proportion of the work during these training years was routine 'service' and only a small proportion of cases had high educational value. This prolonged gestation nevertheless meant that consultant applicants were very experienced; usually with extensive knowledge of several specialist fields and an expertise in research. British doctors were highly regarded and the system seemed to work effectively. Despite its effectiveness, there were several reasons why the old system was discarded and 'structured training' adopted:

- All European Economic Community (EEC) countries have agreed that their professional qualifications should be equivalent. Under European legislation, 'specialist' is the title given to a fully trained doctor. Specialists must hold a CCST and European law states that doctors should be able to obtain their CCST within 6 years of full registration. British apprenticeship training usually took more than 6 years and the system had to be changed to comply with European legislation.
- Apprenticeship training suited doctors pursuing a full-time career in a specialty. However, an increasing proportion of medical graduates want to give priority to their families during certain periods of their life. In theory, structured training allows for these aspirations as it is easier to determine an individual's level of expertise and so allocate a suitable training slot when that doctor returns from a career break.
- The firm-based training system became less satisfactory when junior doctors' hours-of-work were reduced and single consultant firms evolved into clinical teams. Individual consultants found it harder to supervise the progress of their trainees and mechanisms were needed to ensure that all trainees receive adequate advice and assistance.
- British training took much longer than training elsewhere and yet the overseas-trained doctors were just as competent. It was felt that the British system could be more efficient.
- The modern hospital consultant is now expected not only to be effective clinically, but also to acquire the educational and managerial skills dis-

cussed in this book. Adding to the burden of knowledge while shortening the time available for education meant that the revised training system had to be more efficient, and hence structured.

Although structured training has many potential benefits, the concept is new and will take time to become established. There are several problems with the new system:

- The new training system is time-consuming for senior medical staff who have to design and run educational programmes and training assessments
- Many of the recommended training courses are very expensive; no new money has been provided
- The service work still has to be done and an inadequate number of new consultant posts have been created to compensate for the reduction in trainees hours of work
- Many doctors with 2 or 3 years SHO experience in a specialty are finding it hard to get registrar posts as demand for registrar posts in popular specialties outstrips their availability
- Existing consultants are reluctant to change their methods of teaching and working

The transition to the new training system is likely to be difficult. A generation of doctors may be produced who have received neither a lengthy apprenticeship, nor properly structured training. These doctors may find their initial period as a consultant very stressful.

Organization of training

The GMC is the organization that regulates the medical profession. It governs professional standards and has recently been given the power to investigate the competence of doctors whose clinical standards may be unsatisfactory. It sets the undergraduate syllabus and accredits medical schools. The GMC gives full registration to doctors who have performed satisfactorily during their pre-registration house jobs. Post-graduate medical training is organized by several professional bodies working together (Box 3.1). The *regional post-graduate deans* are responsible for supervising the employment and education of PRHOs and SHOs not yet committed to a particular specialty. They also review the progress of specialist registrars. The deans appoint *post-graduate clinical tutors* in each hospital to assist them. The clinical tutors work from the hospital post-graduate centres and are consultant staff or GPs interested in education. They organize teaching courses and provide counselling for PRHOs and SHOs. The *medical royal colleges and specialty faculties* set professional standards for their specialty. They define syllabuses, organize examinations and accredit departments. They are governed by an elected council who appoint *regional educational advisers* and *college tutors* in each hospital. This hierarchy looks after the professional and educational needs of trainees committed to a particular specialty. Both

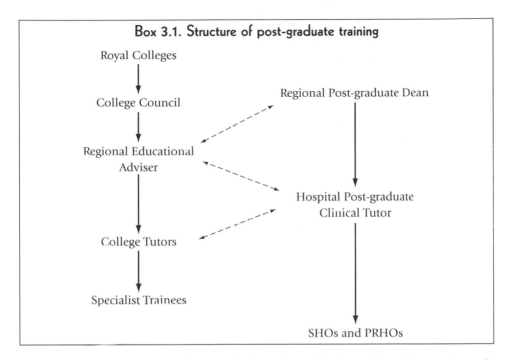

Box 3.1. Structure of post-graduate training

Royal Colleges

College Council

Regional Educational Adviser

College Tutors

Specialist Trainees

Regional Post-graduate Dean

Hospital Post-graduate Clinical Tutor

SHOs and PRHOs

teams should liaise; the mechanism for achieving this will vary in each trust. Each trainee should have a nominated *educational supervisor* who is responsible for ensuring that the trainee is getting a satisfactory education.

The process of training

Box 3.2 summarizes the components of structured training. Each specialty defines its own professional requirements. The object of training is to obtain the *Certificate of Completion of Specialist Training* or CCST. This certificate is recognized throughout the EEC as an indication that a doctor has specialist skills, and in some countries has the additional importance of enabling that doctor to claim specialist fees from insurance or social funds. It is essential that trainees think carefully and take advice before entering a specialty. Once in a specialist registrar post, the opportunities for a change of career will be restricted.

General SHO posts

Before obtaining their specialist registrar post, trainees will spend some time at SHO grade. The initial phase of training, when general skills are acquired and the doctor is undecided about the future has been called the *sump*. The length of time SHOs spend in the sump will depend upon the popularity of the specialty that they seek to enter. Popular specialities will have high entry standards, and the applicants will need to demonstrate broad clinical experience and have a good CV.

Box 3.2. Components of structured training

- Production of an educational syllabus for each period of training
- An indication of the knowledge required to pass each examination
- Advice on what skills a trainee should possess and how these skills can be learned. Some colleges are now making attendance at certain training courses mandatory.
- Annual assessments of progress conducted by the post-graduate dean's office to ensure that each trainee is progressing satisfactorily
- Formative assessments conducted during the year by consultants or college tutors
- Arrangements for trainees to receive advice and assistance from staff not directly responsible for their professional progress (mentoring)
- Mechanisms to help trainees who are failing to progress satisfactorily

---

Specialist SHO posts

Initial specialist training will take place at SHO level, usually for 2 years. Trainees entering a specialty must register with their chosen royal college — and may have to pay for the privilege. Initial professional examinations will be taken as an SHO and must be passed before obtaining a registrar post.

Specialist registrar posts

The specialist registrar is the main training grade. Each training post must be approved by the appropriate royal college and only a limited number of posts, determined according to specialist need anticipated by a committee called AGMETS, will be available. Only training in accredited UK posts will count towards the award of the CCST. Although it will be theoretically possible to obtain a specialist post 6 years after full registration as a doctor, it is likely that trainees in popular specialities will spend considerably longer in training or other sub-consultant posts as they improve their CVs so that they are competitive when applying for desirable consultant posts.

Monitoring progress

Once a trainee enters a specialty they will join a department or training school. In a well-organized rotation he or she will have an induction meeting with the college tutor or educational supervisor who should make clear what is expected of them. Box 3.3 lists some of the topics that might be discussed at this initial meeting. The educational supervisor should then monitor the candidates progress and provide appropriate feedback.

Reviews of progress

Structured training requires the trainee to be reviewed formally each year by the post-graduate dean's office. Reports on progress are received from individual hospitals and trainees must have performed adequately in the preceding year if they are to advance to the next stage of their training.

Box 3.3. Departmental training plan

- A modular plan for developing clinical expertise
- An examination syllabus
- Recommended skills courses that the trainee should attend
- Details of local procedures for personal and skills assessment
- Discussion of local requirements for maintaining log books
- Requirements for written or oral presentations to department or college
- Details of when further informal departmental assessments will take place and an indication of when formal assessments by the dean's office will take place

---

Inevitably some candidates will perform poorly and will not be allowed to proceed. Appeals mechanisms are being established to allow for failures to contest the decision, particularly if problems arise late in their training.

Examinations

Structured training involves a series of formal examinations, which must be passed if the candidate is to progress. The nature and content of these examinations is defined by the royal college responsible for the specialty.

Specialist accreditation

The CCST is awarded by the GMC on the basis of recommendations that it receives from the royal colleges. A CCST is valid throughout Europe, although appropriate registration procedures must be completed which may include a language test and dealing, sometimes at length, with local bureaucracies.

Appraisal and assessment

Terminology

This subject has become confused because authors have used different terms for similar educational processes. In our view:

Appraisal is a process in which trainer and trainee look ahead and plan the next stage of training. A series of measurable targets is established so that the trainee knows what is expected. Advice is given about how these targets can be achieved. Appraisal is an individual process in which consensus is sought between the trainee and their advisor. Some writers use the term formative assessment for this process.

Assessment is a process in which the progress of a trainee is measured against established criteria. The criteria may have been established at a previous appraisal meeting, or may be an examination syllabus. Good assessment mechanisms should be consistent so that candidates can be compared fairly. No consensus between assessor and candidate is necessary. The term summative assessment is sometimes used for to describe formal measurements of progress, usually during examinations.

Throughout training, appraisal and assessment should become cyclical so that each meeting between trainer and trainee both reviews the past and looks towards the future. We know that not everyone will agree with these definitions and if you want to read more about assessment, we recommend that you read *The Good Assessment Guide* (1997), published by the Joint Centre for Education in Medicine, 33 Millman Street, London WC1N 3EJ.

Value of assessment

Assessments can be performed for several reasons (Box 3.4). Educationalists believe that regular appraisal and assessment allows people to make optimum use of their talents and improves the way people are taught. Assessment techniques have been used by the military for many years and have proved effective, but their value in medicine remains unproven. A well-organized highly motivated clinician is unlikely to need much help, but an effective counselling session can draw attention to aspects of career development of which the trainee is unaware.

Box 3.4. Reasons for assessing students

- To judge the acquisition of essential skills and knowledge
- To measure improvements over time
- To rank students
- To diagnose student difficulties
- To evaluate teaching methods
- To evaluate the effectiveness of the course
- To motivate students to study

It is easy for the appraisal/assessment cycle to degenerate into a process which 'must' be done because that is what the educational contract says, but which is of little value to any of the participants. The most important aspects of the process are likely to be the establishment of clear targets, achievable by the majority of trainees, against which the individuals attainments can be measured. Failure to attain these targets will indicate that a trainee is having problems and repeated failure after remedial assistance may indicate that the trainee should look at another career.

Assessments should take place at sensible intervals: typically at the start, mid-point and end of an allocation. Most trainees perform adequately and simply need to be encouraged to concentrate on particular aspects of their career, develop certain skills, or attend useful courses. A few junior trainees are temperamentally unsuited to their chosen career and may soon come to realize it. They may be surprisingly grateful if they can be gently offered the option of moving to another specialty. Assessment meetings are most useful, and also most difficult, when the perceptions of trainee and trainers vary significantly. Handled well the assessment can help to eliminate bad characteristics, but conflicts are always possible.

Assessing a trainee

Assessment interviews are not easy and assessors need to develop the necessary skills. It is best to attend an appropriate course before regularly assessing trainees. Meetings between an educational supervisor and a trainee should be held in a quiet place where the conversation cannot be overheard. Assessment meetings should not be hurried, interrupted or too informal.

A trainer should prepare for the interview by looking at the trainee's past records and the most recent training plan to see whether targets have been met. Obtain opinions from everyone who has worked with the trainee. This can be done informally, but if the report is critical, for instance on interpersonal skills, it is desirable to have written evidence to support statements. Many specialties have developed assessment tools to assist the process. Some departments ask their trainees to assess themselves and discrepancies between the trainee's and the supervisor's views of progress are particularly worth exploring.

Process of assessment

The trainee must be clear about the nature of the session. Sessions involving appraisal and assessment of professional progress are not confidential. Indeed the conclusions of the discussions should be documented and a copy held in the trainee's records. Confidential personal counselling should not normally take place at an assessment session unless both parties agree to some of the discussions being 'off the record'. The assessor is key to this process. Box 3.5 indicates the characteristics that are required. Box 3.6 lists the objectives of an effective meeting.

Box 3.5. Characteristics of a good assessor

- Listens
- Reflects back the trainee's comments when appropriate so that there can be detailed discussions of aspects of concern to the trainee
- Actively supports the trainee's decisions when they are appropriate
- Arranges counselling when needed (see below)
- Judges progress positively rather than emphasizing criticism
- Informs trainees of opinions expressed on progress without censoring
- Identifies needs

Box 3.6. Results of an effective session

- Gives feedback to the trainee on performance, discussing those aspects of career development that are going well and pinpointing aspects which need to improve
- Reviews what progress the trainee has made towards previously established targets
- Reviews the trainee's logbook to see if clinical training has been adequate
- Results in a mutually agreed plan of action for the next training period
- Decides an appropriate time for the next review
- Ends with a copy of the professional evaluation and list of agreed targets being given to the trainee

While most assessment meetings are straightforward, a few can be very stressful for both participants. The truth can hurt and in medicine we are not used to brutally honest discussions of our ability. Until the whole process becomes better integrated into the medical career structure it is inevitable that some people will leave an appraisal session downhearted by being criticized, even if the adverse comments formed only a small portion of the appraisal. Curiously the most difficult sessions are usually the most useful in the long term, as confronting people when they have difficulties enables them to tackle problems that they are aware of, but have put to one side. Criticism should always be combined with positive suggestions and a sensible action plan agreed. Assessment is a two-way process and a trainer ought to listen to a trainee's criticisms of their educational programme so that each can discuss why difficulties have occurred and any weak aspects of the course can be improved.

Being assessed

Most doctors are unfamiliar with continuous professional development. For the foreseeable future, the quality of assessors will vary. As a trainee you should prepare for an assessment session by making sure that your logbook is up-to-date, and should decide how your progress compares with your peers. If you want to criticize some aspect of your training you should try to gather evidence to justify your statements. Some department use self-assessment tools. If you are asked to fill in an appraisal document, try to return it to your educational supervisor quickly.

Go into the meeting with an open mind and listen to all that is said. Do not be too upset by criticism, listen to all the advice that is given, do not just focus on one aspect. When future targets are discussed make sure that they seem sensible. It is better to reject or alter a target at this stage than to fail to achieve it in 6 months time. Finally, remember that most people moan about the present regime, even if everything else is likely to be worse, and that there are few 'quick-fixes' in a big organization, so forgive your assessor if not all your problems can be solved.

The difficult trainee

Typical problems include trainees:

- Who repeatedly fail exams
- Whose self-assessment varies markedly from others' opinion of them
- Who consistently fail to take advice or reach pre-arranged targets
- Who are unsuited to a particular career

It is essential that the appraisal meetings with these trainees are properly documented. Remedial training targets should be agreed, documented and signed. If a trainee is likely to disagree with their assessments, written evidence from a variety of sources should be available to support the supervisor's reports. This evidence may be needed at an appeal tribunal if the training contract is eventually terminated. It is sometimes advisable to involve a second senior doctor in the interviews to ensure that there is a witness to proceedings.

Formal reviews of progress

Trainees will have a formal annual review of progress by the dean's office. These reviews are designed to ensure that unsuitable trainees do not progress to specialist status. Hopefully, trainees will not receive unexpected surprises at these meetings as departmental counselling should enable trainees to understand how well they are thought to be progressing.

Continuing professional development

As the concept of assessment and appraisal becomes better established, it may, as in other industries and professions, become a process that continues through ones career, with periodic assessment of personal training needs compared to organizational requirements.

Counselling

The dictionary definition of counselling is: *advice given formally; to assist or guide*. Counselling includes the professional appraisal and assessment mechanisms described above, but the term is more commonly used to mean personal counselling. A doctor may need counselling for reasons such as a failure to integrate into a department, emotional or financial stress, or poor examination or interview performance. Particular help may need to be offered to someone who feels they are suffering harassment at work. Most commonly though, counselling is sought by doctors who want to plan their career.

Personal counselling

Personal counselling is usually best provided by someone with no direct professional responsibility for the trainee. Hospitals should have a mechanism, which the trainees know about, to deal with personal problems. It is generally best to avoid giving off-the-cuff advice, but instead plan to meet for a specified length of time in a quiet place where confidentiality can be assured. This should be arranged when pagers and telephones can safely be left with a secretary so that there will be no interruptions. By making the proceedings formal, the trainee can be assured that he or she is being taken seriously and that the best possible advice is being offered. At the outset a 'contract' should be formed between the counsellor and visitor. This should include discussion of:

- The topics that the discussion will cover
- The duration of the session
- Whether written records will be kept
- Whether the counsellor will give personal opinions, or those of a group of assessors
- Whether anyone will made aware of the contents of the discussions

Counselling sessions

Counselling can be exceptionally difficult, particularly for doctors who are used to structuring their time rigidly in order to gain the maximum information from a brief encounter with a patient. Senior doctors are prone to lead the conversation, forcing their opinions on a trainee who may have had a different agenda in mind. A good counsellor will let the trainee talk, but encourage them by making judicious comments to move towards working out for themselves what they want. Ideally, it is only after discovering how the trainee views things that the counsellor comments. Although trainees may appear to want firm advice, it is safer to list all the options with their relevant advantages and drawbacks, rather than going straight for a single option. Ultimately the trainee must make up their own mind and be sure about it, otherwise they will, possibly correctly, blame their advisor for future failings. Sometimes, the counsellor may feel that the problem exceeds their own skills and may suggest that the trainee or colleague seeks advice elsewhere. A list of sources of help is given in Chapter 2.

Mentoring

A mentor is defined as a *wise counsellor*. Some educationalists support the concept that all students should have a *mentor*, who is there to guide the student through the educational programme. A mentor is an educational supervisor with the skills described in the previous section, but who should additionally provide support to the trainee in areas outside the purely professional and educational aspects of their life. An effective mentor should be able to influence and guide his or her protégés in a way that they find constructive and yet unobtrusive. Anyone with a little bit of training, appropriate knowledge and the ability to relate to others can act as a mentor although it is likely that both senior and trainee will be in the same line of work and thus able to understand each other's difficulties.

The key to effective mentoring is that a rapport should develop between the two people involved. Mentors are unlikely to be effective if they are imposed on a student as there is no guarantee that the two personalities will relate. Many students never feel the need to seek assistance or, if they do, naturally seek out colleagues for advice without consciously giving the process a name. Mentors serve a particularly useful role if the junior perceives themselves to be a member of a minority group struggling to achieve a goal and the mentor is a member of the same group who has already reached the goal. Mentoring is better performed informally in a pub or over a meal, rather than the formal setting of an appraisal/assessment or counselling session.

In scientific research the mentor of a research student is expected not only to ensure that the student understands what is expected of them and to ensure that they are making progress with their investigations, but should also ensure that they understand the ethics of science: what is acceptable practice, what constitutes fraudulently produced results, and what are unacceptable ways to publish findings.

When acting as a mentor, it is usually advisable to remain impartial and adopt a passive rather than active advisory role. However, there may be times to be more proactive and, for instance, act as intermediary if the relationship between a trainee and those around is under strain or has broken down. Not all students progress successfully through the stages of educational development required as undergraduates or post-graduates. Just because a trainee has performed well in the past does not mean that external circumstances or stresses cannot affect future achievements. A mentor should be someone the trainee can seek out for help or advice. Sadly, those most in need of help are often those least able to seek it for themselves, and one should not be afraid to offer assistance if you suspect that someone is under stress.

Mentoring networks

There are mentoring networks within the medical profession, but you have to look hard to find them. The idea of mentoring is not well established in the medical community, which probably reflects lack of time or staff to do it, rather than lack of support for the idea. A mentoring network should enable those people who have mentoring responsibility to get together and discuss the different aspects of mentoring, to learn how to provide help and to gain some experience in the skills required to become a mentor. Such links may help to solve problems mentors come across, as well as increase their own network of helpful links.

Related topics

Stress (p. 19)
Advice (p. 20)

4. TEACHING AND LEARNING

Objectives of this section
- to understand how people learn
- to organize and chair a teaching session
- to help you work effectively for examinations

Medical education is a hot topic. Since the Calman report in 1992 there has been enormous concern about the way we teach and assess medical trainees. The reduction in hours and years of training has led to anxieties about whether educational standards can be maintained. Structured teaching of theory does not necessarily mean that trainees have been adequately prepared to practice medicine, which requires a high level of practical skills together with elements of experience and wisdom.

People learn, and teachers inspire, in different ways. Individuals respond differently to written, visual, aural and electronic teaching methods, and favour different styles of teaching. Interactive small group teaching gives trainees a better understanding of principles than didactic lectures. Practical skills are best learned by practice. Self-directed and problem-based learning, in which the pupils decide for themselves what they want to investigate, works well for some. Any method of teaching can be effective, but all will fail if the course structure is badly organized, the teachers uninspiring, or the students use inappropriate methods of learning.

Effective teaching and learning require effort and enthusiasm. It is almost impossible to prove that one teaching method is better than another. What may appear a fad to one student may be inspirational to another. Most doctors have never been taught to teach, and doctors are usually sceptical of new educational techniques. Many use a didactic teaching style which emphasizes facts about clinical conditions, but does not explain the underlying principles. As a result, many students adopt a passive style of learning, expecting facts to be given to them and not seeking knowledge for themselves. Teachers must improve the way they teach and assess trainees, while trainees must take greater responsibility for their education.

Learning techniques

The way we learn changes with age. Young children memorize information as a series of unconnected facts. As they grow older, improved motor skills and previous experiences enable problems to be tackled and facts memorized in a more logical fashion. Eventually knowledge is consolidated into a series of principles which can then be applied to any new situation.

Types of learning

There are several different ways of learning (Box 4.1).

Box 4.1. Characteristics of different ways of learning

Surface learners	Deep learners	Strategic learners
Motivated by fear of failure	Motivated by interest in subject	Competitive — motivated to achieve high grades
Good rote learners with good memories	Seek to understand	Patchy knowledge of facts and understanding
Learn facts without principles	Questioning	List makers
Minds organized to promote recall rather than understanding	Wary of generalizations — doubt conclusions	Use algorithms
Poor understanding of basic principles	Favour self-directed learning	Knowledge organized for quick-fix
More dependent on tutors and course material		Limited clinical reasoning

In practice, people use each of these learning styles at times and according to their needs.

Students with a *surface approach to learning* have retentive memories. They are able to recall facts quickly, but do not catalogue or organize their knowledge. People who are good at surface learning perform well in general knowledge quizzes, but have a poor understanding of underlying principles and are not good at analysing or interpreting data.

Students with a *deep approach to learning* try to understand the concepts underlying a subject. Understanding the principles then allows them to set about solving problems or answering examination questions.

A third group are termed *strategic* learners. These students adopt a variety of learning styles designed to reach a particular goal with the minimum effort. They cram knowledge and use crib sheets to prepare for anticipated examination questions. There is evidence that students who adopt this style of learning perform badly in the long-term, and that their knowledge is patchy and poorly retained.

Typically, during schooling up to the mid-teens, pupils use the surface approach. Good teaching ought to encourage a shift in mental processes and most students ought to be 'deep' learning by the time they enter university. However, because they have to learn so many facts, medical students are likely to continue surface learning for longer. Some retain this approach until they are faced with their advanced professional examinations. Well-designed examinations require candidates to understand principles rather than simply regurgitate facts. Some trainees find it difficult to make the transition to deep learning so late in their careers. Undergraduate courses are changing, so that more effective methods of learning are encouraged.

It is worth analysing the way you learn as there are considerable advantages to adopting the deep approach. Box 4.2 indicates the benefits of making an effort to understand a subject rather than just learning the facts.

Box 4.2. Benefits of a deep approach to learning

- Fewer dissociated facts need to be memorized
- You are less likely to feel overburdened with knowledge
- Learning becomes easier and more enjoyable
- Knowledge is retained longer
- It is easier to revise
- Principles can be transferred from one field of study to another
- You develop an ability to analyse and question, and can then initiate research in fields where knowledge is lacking

---

Personal factors influencing learning

The effectiveness with which you learn will be influenced by factors such as those in Box 4.3.

Box 4.3. Factors influencing learning

- The structure and perceived relevance of the course
- The related educational goals such as continuous appraisal or examinations. Multiple choice questionnaire (MCQ) exams, for example, demand a higher proportion of rote learning
- The amount of thought that you give to how you plan to achieve your educational targets
- Your interest in the topics under discussion
- Social factors that interfere with study time or motivation, for instance personal relationships or hobbies
- Psychological factors such as anxiety, depression or stress

---

You have greater control over these factors than you might think. When beginning a course, ask around to find out what course books are available.

For example, in physiology there are a several good texts for post-graduate examinations, but candidates have individual preferences. Spend time choosing one you like. Set aside time each day for study and ensure that you can work without interruption. Plan regular breaks so that you concentrate when you are studying, but still have time for relaxation. Take advantage of any courses or tutorials that are available, having others around you who are also facing the same challenges helps.

Other factors influencing learning

Other factors which influence the way you learn are:

- The way you are taught
- Where you are taught

You can nowadays learn in many different ways: by lectures or tutorials, by reading books, watching TV or video, or by computer-aided learning (CAL).

As a student you may not be able to improve your teacher's performance (although appraisal forms allow you some feedback), but you can help yourself understand. Box 4.4 suggests obvious ways to help yourself learn. If you have had problems learning in the past, find out if there is a study skills course you could attend. Such courses can improve your ability to organize knowledge, manage your time and read quickly. If you cannot attend a course, obtain a book on this subject.

Box 4.4. Improving learning during classes

- Listen and try to make sense of key information as the speaker talks
- Avoid compulsive note-taking if this means that you do not listen
- If you lose track, make a positive effort to concentrate. A well-structured talk will offer opportunities to get back into the subject
- In a small group, speak up if you do not understand something. Get the teacher to recap or re-phrase what has been said
- Try not to be distracted by the lecturer's mannerisms, failures in the A-V material, bluebottles, or fantasies about the student sitting in front of you

---

Social and environmental factors may be under your control. Lack of sleep, alcohol, a recent big meal, extremes of temperature, noise and uncomfortable clothing all reduce your ability to concentrate. Some people learn best early in the day, others late at night. Plan your work schedule appropriately.

Why learn to teach?

Often people recognize that a few charismatic teachers have influenced the way that they think. In contrast, a teacher's failure to capture and maintain his pupils interest will mean that they do not learn and lose interest in the topic. Doctors should try to pass on their knowledge and enthusiasms to others by being good communicators.

Traditional didactic medical teaching can be rather drab. Lectures or poorly run tutorials are soporific. The concept of 'microsleep' is well recognized; typically students lose concentration every 15 minutes when passively learning. This interval can be even shorter for students in the medical profession (as little as 5 minutes!). Bad teaching is a waste of everyone's time and you should try to improve your skills.

Small group teaching

Soon after qualification you make the transition from pupil to teacher. Initially you have to teach medical students, later you are asked to teach your peers. Formal lecture presentations are discussed elsewhere, this section is about 'interactive small group discussion', a term which includes tutorials, seminars, discussion groups and problem-based learning sessions. Well-conducted tutorials and seminars are more effective than lectures because students and teachers interact, and a deep rather than superficial approach to a subject can be taught. Questions can be asked and confusing issues clarified as soon as they arise.

Whatever the actual format of small group teaching, the principles of organization are similar. A successful small group teaching session requires:

- Preparation
- A lively and questioning group of students
- Feedback

The roles of the tutor leading a group are to:

- Manage the learning task — making the task challenging rather than boring
- Manage individual learners — giving feedback and clarifying concepts
- Manage the educational process — ensuring the syllabus is covered and that candidates are given feedback about their performance

Preparation is the key to success.

Preparation

Group size
There is no correct number for a small group although 8–12 is probably about right. Most often the group size is determined not by the teacher but by the number of trainees who are studying for a particular exam and are free to attend. If a big group has to be subdivided for teaching, try to mix personality types so that each tutorial group has its share of extrovert as well as shy characters.

The location
Book a comfortable room with appropriate space and seating for everyone. Seat people in a circle to encourage them to become involved. Discourage

distractions; secretaries should answer telephones and bleeps and only interrupt the tutorial if it is essential. Niceties such as coffee or tea, especially at the beginning or the end of the day, help to revitalize people and provide a relaxed atmosphere while people congregate, but should never interrupt teaching once it has started.

Learning aids
Clean the whiteboard or make sure that the flip chart has plenty of paper; check that the pens work. Ensure that the overhead and slide projectors and video equipment are available if needed. Book extra equipment such as mannikins well in advance. Make sure everything is working before the teaching session is due to start.

Information
Make sure everyone knows where and when they are meeting and the subject of the tutorial. Start and finish on time.

Teacher preparation
Know your subject; read up if necessary. Identify key learning targets relevant to your group. Some targets will require a factual understanding of a topic, but other goals might be the development of communication skills and critical thinking. Then consider how to teach these and how to develop the discussions. Different small group teaching styles include:

- The mini-lecture
- Problem- or scenario-based discussions
- Question-and-answer sessions
- Student-led discussion

Select the most appropriate approach for the main part of your session, but bear in mind that a mixture of styles is desirable as different students learn in different ways. You may wish to prepare visual aids, handouts or reference lists.

Student preparation
You will be able to achieve more in a teaching session if the students have some basic knowledge of the subject beforehand. However, trainees generally turn up with different degrees of knowledge and understanding. You might consider starting the teaching session with a question sheet or problem-based task that takes 10 minutes or so and helps the students identify what they already know. When leading a series of tutorials you should finish each session by explaining what you plan to cover next time, so that students can do some reading.

Group dynamics
The style the teacher adopts is often dictated by the format of the session. Mini-lectures and seminars inevitably involve the teacher more than the student, whereas problem-based scenarios or free discussion groups are stu-

dent- rather than teacher-led. In student-led sessions, the tutor should encourage, and control the direction of discussions, but not dominate proceedings or provide all the information. It is important to get everyone involved and maintain a momentum so that people feel that the discussions are moving towards their goals.

Groups, whether they are tutorial groups with an educational task or committees charged with a management job, show the five stages listed in Box 4.5. As you work with small groups you will come to understand these interactions and be able to encourage the transition from disorganization into action and achievement.

Box 4.5. Stages in group interaction

- **Forming** — members get to know each other
- **Storming** — they establish their roles within the group and aim to establish a dominance
- **Norming** — people get on with the job
- **Performing** — the group hopefully achieves it objectives
- **Adjourning** — the group concludes its task and looks towards disbanding

---

Feedback

We all like to be praised for our work, but feedback cannot always be positive. Evaluation of your individual teaching sessions may be informative, particularly if you are trying out new styles of teaching, or a new topic. Informal feedback using questions such as 'Was there anything you didn't understand?' or 'Was the way we approached the subject useful?' may help you find out whether you taught well. If you prefer anonymous feedback you should design a suitable assessment form and distribute it at the start of the session.

Feedback is essential when you are supervising a tutorial group for several weeks. Interaction between members of a group and their teacher varies and a teaching style that worked well in the past may be disliked by another group of students. Modify your style to suit. The relationship between trainee and teacher will change with time as people relax and this may also influence the value and honesty of their comments. Most important of all, learning should be fun!

Problem-based learning

Several medical schools have adopted a 'problem-based learning' syllabus. Students learn in groups of up to 12 which meet once or twice a week. The course tutor provides a series of problems for the students to consider. Apart from explaining any technical terms and ensuring that the group is interacting effectively, the tutor then remains in the background, possibly directing the groups thoughts by an occasional question, but not otherwise teaching directly. The group has to organize itself and set about solving the problem before its next meeting. It is taught to use a staged process: the *'seven jump'* (Box 4.6).

Box 4.6. The 'seven-jump' in problem-based learning

1. Unknown terms and concepts are clarified
2. The problems that the question raises must be discovered and debated
3. The problems must be understood and explained
4. The explanations must be arranged so that a coherent description of the process can be produced
5. The group must formulate learning-goals
6. Gaps in knowledge must be filled by seeking information from papers, books or experts
7. The knowledge must be integrated into a comprehensive and complete solution which is understood by the whole group. Sources of information must be quoted.

The key to problem-based learning is the questions that are asked. They must be unambiguous and direct the students towards gaining knowledge in the required fields. Topics must build upon each other, so that learning takes place in an appropriate series of challenges. The medical schools using this method of education have moved away from specialty-based learning to a broader-based syllabus.

Problem-based learning has its enthusiastic advocates. They claim it encourages a deep approach to learning and helps develop a life-long learning habit. Students take time to adapt to this type of education, and cannot be assessed properly by traditional medical examinations. There is evidence that graduates of problem-based courses retain information longer, but there is no evidence that they become better or more effective doctors.

Conclusion

The Hippocratic oath (Chapter 13, p. 156) includes the concept that all doctors should pass on knowledge to their successors. British hospital consultants have teaching included within their job descriptions. Not all doctors are good teachers and some are dreadful. Teaching requires time, organization, knowledge and enthusiasm. Educational courses are being established to help doctors teach, and educating the teachers should help to improve standards.

Preparing for examinations

Examinations are a hurdle designed to ensure that the standards of training are maintained. Preparing for an examination is not just about learning facts and understanding principles, it is also about presenting knowledge in a satisfactory fashion to the examiner.

The examination

The techniques used for summative assessment, that is examination of candidates, are listed in Box 4.7. Identify how you will be assessed. The examination department of your college or faculty should send you a syllabus, but some syllabuses are vague, and you may need to get additional advice from your college tutor or recent successful candidates. Each type of assessment requires different skills. Practice is essential; your knowledge and confidence will grow and you will be able to correct your weaknesses.

Box 4.7. Techniques used for summative assessment

- Essays
- Short answers
- Multiple choice questions
- Clinical examinations
- Objectively structured clinical examinations (OSCEs)
- Vivas, which may be structured (objectively structured oral examinations, OSOEs)
- Review of course work, or logbooks
- Dissertations or theses

Types of examination

Medical examinations used to consist of essays, vivas and clinical examinations. Fairer and more appropriate ways of testing knowledge are being introduced.

Essays

Essays are a traditional method of examination. They are relatively easy to set, but labour intensive to mark, and it is difficult to ensure consistent marking between different examiners. Only a limited number of topics can be covered in one exam paper, and results are influenced by the writing skills of the candidate.

Short answers

Short answers with examiners comparing answers with mark sheets, provide better consistency and enable more topics to be covered. Candidates must state as many facts as possible in each answer and allocate equal time to answering each section.

MCQs

MCQs test a wide range of factual knowledge quickly. Computer marking ensures accurate and reproducible results, but unless the papers are extremely well designed, they encourage surface learning of facts.

Vivas

These are notoriously difficult for some candidates, who cannot cope with the pressure of the examination despite performing adequately at work. Structured vivas, in which every candidate is asked similar questions, may eliminate some of the unfairness perceived to have occurred in the past.

Clinical examinations

The classic format begins with a long case, during which the candidate completes a history and clinical examination before seeing the examiners; and is then questioned. The long case is followed by a series of short clinical cases, during which the candidate is expected to recognize a series of physical signs. There is a considerable element of luck in these examinations, as the performance of the candidate is influenced by whether they recognize the, often rare, conditions of the patients and are able to elicit the appropriate physical signs. Nowadays, in an attempt to make this type of examination fairer, scoring sheets are used and the candidate is observed throughout the long-case.

Objective structured clinical examinations (OSCEs)

Candidates are observed performing practical tasks at a series of skill stations. Examples include interpretation of X-rays or laboratory results, and tests of life support skills. There is greater emphasis on interpretation of data, while the use of manikins and simulated patients have made the results of OSCEs more reproducible than the old-style clinical examination.

Course work

Some examinations require you to produce a logbook, series of case commentaries or a dissertation. Try to keep your logbook up-to-date, searching for information about old cases just before an examination is a stress you can do without. Hospital information systems can provide a lifeline if you are in trouble. Beg assistance from someone who can use the hospital computers. If you have to produce a dissertation, read the regulations carefully and keep to the required format. Typing, printing and binding take time, so don't leave them to the last minute.

In summary, examiners are trying to improve the way in which trainees are assessed, to recognize the limitations of the examination process and to eradicate examiner bias.

Passing examinations

Essays

Essays must be planned. Your aim is to prove that you have understood the question by presenting the relevant facts concisely, unambiguously and logically. Begin by reading the precise wording of the question. The stem of the question might for instance begin: 'Discuss', 'Compare and contrast' or 'How would you'; and each stem requires a different style of answer. Spend a couple of minutes jotting down your thoughts on the subject on scrap paper. Although it may appear a waste of precious writing time, this planning period allows you to concentrate on the question and organize your answer efficiently. It also provides you with space to note ideas that may occur to you while writing the essay. If you run seriously short of time for your last question, submitting an essay plan will often score higher marks than trying to write prose in a rush.

Candidates who omit the planning stage frequently miss the point of the question and instead randomly write all they know about a subject. You risk losing marks if the examiner has to plough through unnecessary information while seeking relevant arguments. Candidates should be cautious about expressing personal attitudes and opinions in essays: the examiner looks for accepted practice. Spend equivalent time on each answer. If your handwriting is difficult to read you can improve its legibility by writing on alternate lines, underlining or using colour to improve clarity.

Short questions

Although your answers will be briefer, the principles of good essay writing apply — correct, logical and organized thought. Watch the clock closely and do not allow yourself to overrun on any individual topic. Each answer, however good, will only score a certain number of marks, but failure to answer a question will usually result in failure of the examination.

The MCQ

The style of MCQs varies, but they are usually phrased for the answers True, False or Don't Know. MCQs may be marked negatively. Negative marking means that a mark is deducted for every wrong answer. This has important implications because you will lose marks if you guess blindly. There are many books and CAL packages which enable you to practise MCQ questions, and these will allow you to analyse the way you answer questions — from knowledge, an educated guess or pure guesswork — and equate this to your results. You can assess whether it will gain or lose you marks if you make 'educated guesses'.

The pass mark of a MCQ examination depends both upon the validity of the questions asked, and the performance of the entrants. Computer analysis of the performance of the current candidates in certain key questions is compared with previous cohorts and the pass mark selected on this basis. As no one knows this information until the examination is over, the only safe policy is to answer all the questions you know and then guess those in which you think you have a reasonable chance of success. Leave other questions unanswered. If you know enough you will pass, and if you do not, you will not.

Keep an eye on the clock, and allow yourself some time for checking at the end. Always read the stem of each question carefully so that you do not misunderstand the meaning of the question. Some people prefer to fill in answers on the question sheet and then transfer them to the computer answer card, but if you use this strategy make sure you transpose accurately. Finally, remember to take your good luck charm!

Vivas

Medicine involves verbal communication skills and the ability to work under pressure; the viva examination tests these characteristics. Both knowledge and presentation are crucial. Most candidates find viva examinations frightening. In the past some examiners delighted in humiliating weak examination candidates. This was inexcusable.

It is essential that you practice viva technique. Your aim should be to answer each question quickly and clearly. In a structured viva the examiner expects the candidate to discuss a number of key points and marks are awarded according to the number of topics completed successfully. Lengthy explanations score few marks. If you do not understand a question, ask the examiner to rephrase it.

Learn to organize your answers so that you present your information in a logical fashion. 'Coathangers' for your answers might include those in Box 4.8. Other 'coathangers' can be invented for ECGs, X-rays, pathological specimens and many other subjects. Make up your own and invent ways of remembering them, even under stress.

Box 4.8. Structures for answering viva questions

Drugs	Trade and generic name, uses, chemical structure, presentation, main action, mode of action, route of administration, dose, indications effects, side-effects, toxicity, kinetics, elimination, special points
Clinical	General appearance, skin, CVS, RS, GI, liver, renal, neurology, endocrine, locomotor, syndromes
Resuscitation	Self-protection, help, airway, breathing, circulation, etc.

Arrive at the exam early so that you are not flustered. Dress tidily. In the examination room concentrate on the examiner who is asking you the questions and try to ignore everyone else. You may use paper to illustrate points that you wish to make. Appear confident. Even if you think you know better, try not to argue with the examiners as you will not score marks for doing so! Some examiners use encouraging body language, others just sit passively. It is extremely difficult to judge how well you have done in a viva, because a good examiner will always try to discover the limits of your knowledge and these may be restricted or extensive. Above all, if you have several vivas in a day and think that you have done poorly in the first, do not give up and get drunk at lunch time. You may have done much better than you thought.

OSCEs

Objectively structured clinical examinations require you to organize your thoughts in a similar way to vivas. Most colleges with an OSCE will tell you the type of tests that their exam contains. Familiar skills will be tested, and you must demonstrate not only that you can have the skill, but that you perform it properly. For instance make sure that you indicate that defibrillators are switched on, and check any bag of 'blood' that you are handed to ensure that the unit is correctly cross-matched for the 'patient'. You must get a pass mark at certain skill stations such as basic and advanced life support techniques if you are to pass the examination.

Related topics

Appraisal and assessment (p. 29)
Talks and lectures (p. 67)
Time management (p. 15)

5. COMPUTERS AND INFORMATION TECHNOLOGY

Objectives of this section

- to understand common computing terms
- to know the various types of computer program you require to do a job
- to realize the benefits and limitations of computers in health care
- to perform a simple information search

Some people get great pleasure from computers' ability to perform many complex and varied tasks; others regard them as antisocial irritants which often work erratically and inefficiently. Computers and their associated programs are complex. Buying a computer does not mean that you will be able to produce anything with it; much time must be invested in learning to use the machine before it will increase your productivity. This learning period is frustrating. Until you are a good typist, computers are unlikely to save time on everyday tasks that you previously did using paper and pencil, although they will allow you to undertake complicated tasks such as editing theses and papers, data analysis, and the production of high quality visual aids more efficiently. The best way to learn about computers is to have a good reason to use one, and the skill sections in this book suggest suitable tasks for you to try.

Computers consists of *hardware*, that is the electrical and mechanical parts of the machine, and *software* which is the digital program that makes the computer work.

Computer hardware

A desktop computer has five groups of components, which may be separate or built into a single box (Box 5.1).

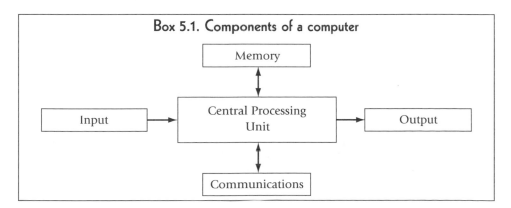

Box 5.1. Components of a computer

Memory

Input → Central Processing Unit → Output

Communications

Central processing unit

The central processing unit (CPU) is the part of the computer that manipulates information. At its heart is a microprocessor which is really just an extremely complicated linkage of electronic switches. The most popular series of microprocessors has been the Intel x86/Pentium range, found in so-called IBM or PC-compatibles, but other manufacturers such as Motorola and Digital also produce CPUs for desktop computers. The power of a computer is governed by the *complexity* of the microprocessor, the *clock-speed* in MHz at which the microprocessor cycles and the number of simultaneous calculations that can be performed (*the addressing*). Up to the mid-1990s desk top computers could perform only one task at a time, but developments in technology now allow *multi-tasking*: several jobs such as printing, word-processing, and communications run simultaneously. Word-processing, and the simple mathematics of accountancy calculations, do not require fast CPUs. However, the manipulation of colour images requires far more powerful processors, and the markets desire for improved graphics and better games encourages manufacturers to produce increasingly powerful computers.

The abilities of a computer are enhanced by a series of *cards* that supplement the CPU. Sound, vision and video cards give multimedia abilities. Most personal computers bought in the high street will be able to play back sound and show moving pictures, but business machines usually lack these abilities.

Memory

The basic element of computing is the binary digit or *bit* which can have the values 0 or 1. A sequence of eight binary bits allows the expression of decimal values from 0 to 255; such a sequence is known as a *byte*. These 255 binary numbers provide the basic language of computing and each number can be allocated to represent a lower or upper case character, a number, a symbol, punctuation or a computer control command. A common sequence is the American standard code for information interchange (*ASCII*). One million bytes is a *megabyte* (MB) and one thousand million bytes is a *gigabyte* (GB). This book in digital form contains about one megabyte of script, while one A4 sized full colour picture requires 40 megabytes to code it.

There are two types of computer memory: stored memory, and electronic random access memory (RAM). Programs are loaded from stored memory into RAM, and from there are fed into the central processor to control calculations. Data loaded from keyboards, disks, scanners or other devices are also held in the RAM until saved elsewhere. RAM is transient; any digital information held in the RAM will be irretrievably lost if there is a power cut, or the computer *crashes* — which means that it ceases to function because of a conflict between instructions within its programs. For this reason it is essential that you regularly *backup* your work into stored memory.

Digital information can be stored permanently using magnetic or optical techniques. Magnetic techniques store information on *digital tape cassettes*, on *floppy disks* or on the much higher capacity *hard drives* supplied with modern computers. A typical floppy disk stores 1.4 MB of information, while hard disk drives currently hold up to a few gigabytes. Optical tape systems and compact disk-read only memory (CD-ROM) laser disks store much greater amounts of information — a typical CD-ROM contains 800 MB, with newer formats such as *digital versatile disks* (DVDs) increasing the amount of stored information to 8 GB or more. Optical, CD and DVD memory cannot be overwritten and is termed *ROM* (read only memory). Hospital clinical information systems may store data on write-once, read many (*WORM*) drives which allow retrieval of data, but are tamper-proof. Information stored on hard and floppy disks is unaffected by power cuts but can be damaged or destroyed by strong magnetic fields. Optical memory stores are more durable. Damage, theft or accident can destroy any store of digital information and you should always make two or three copies of important documents and store them separately.

Input devices

Most current computers are controlled by *keyboards* and your ability to use a computer depends greatly on your skill as a typist. Voice input and control systems are being developed. They require fast computers with large memories, but may become an aid to poor typists. *Mice* and the trackerpads are an intuitive way to control computers, but are a slow way to input data. Scanners allow images to be converted to digital form, and in combination with optical character recognition (OCR) software can convert written text to digital form so that it can be entered into a word processing program. *Optical mark readers* (OMRs) enable information on forms, such as MCQ answer sheets, to be transferred rapidly to a computer. Freehand drawing images can be fed into a computer from a pressure sensitive drawing tablet such as those manufactured by Wacom™. *Bar code readers* can be used to identify patients and match them with their records.

Output devices

The most obvious output device from a computer is the *monitor* screen which may be monochrome, grey scale or be able to output in 16,256, thousands or millions of colours. *Printers* may also be black and white, or coloured. Older printers used typewriter technology which involved a moving head with pistons on it stamping through an ink ribbon, but these dot matrix printers have been superseded by ink jet and laser technology. The definition of the resulting print is defined by the resolution of the printing head: at least 600 dots per inch (dpi) is now standard. The computer output may also be fed into *electronic* or *fax* links, for rapid transmission of data, or stored on floppy disks which can be sent by mail.

Communications

Personal computers can be linked through a telephone network by using a *modem* which encodes digital information for transmission to another computer or fax machine. Domestic telephone lines transmit data relatively slowly as the modem has to translate the data into an analogue signal before it can be transmitted. Commercial organizations use high speed digital phone lines to communicate over long distances; but the line rental is expensive. Optical cable systems, laid around one site allow almost instantaneous communication between individual personal computers and integrate the individual desktop computers into a single system. Computers can be linked to other medical equipment to control function and analyse results.

The Internet

The Internet links a huge number of computers into a single world-wide network. To join the Internet, you need a computer, a modem and a *service provider*. The service provider supplies you with appropriate communications software and a telephone number for your modem to ring. Your modem links with the service providers' computer and can communicate anywhere in the world for the price of a local telephone call. The Internet consists of three main parts: e-mail, usenet and the World Wide Web. The Web has expanded phenomenally in the second half of the 1990s and its ultimate potential is still unclear. Some people's lives have been transformed by instantaneous, cheap global communications, others manage quite satisfactorily without knowing anything about it!

Buying yourself a computer

The technology changes so rapidly that it is impossible to offer firm advice. However, certain factors remain consistent as technology changes. A computer ought to have each of the five components so far discussed. A £150–250 ink-jet printer is now neat and reliable, so there is little point in spending more on an expensive laser printer if your purchase is for personal use. £250–350 monitors are adequate, only buy a big monitor if you plan to work a lot with graphics. Stored memory is cheap and you will not save a lot by skimping. Get the biggest hard disk you can afford as it is likely to fill up as you buy more programs. The difficult decision comes in trying to decide how much RAM to buy and what type of CPU. With these two items cost and capability are roughly proportional. Last year's computer will be out of date in 2 years, while this year's model will be out of date in 3 years! As this year's model (Box 5.2) is likely to be twice the cost of last year's, you have to make a personal trade-off of the benefits. Whatever you buy, its value has halved by the time you have left the store! Expensive multimedia computers now include features such as telephone answering, hi-fi sound and digital TV with video-editing capabilities. These appeal to enthusiasts, but the complexity of such machines makes them harder to understand and more prone to software crashes. Bear in mind that if all you want to do is word-processing, you would be better off buying a simple dedicated word-processor.

Box 5.2. Specification for typical 1997 computer

233 MHz CPU, 32-bit addressing
32 MB RAM
Video and sound card
4 GB Hard disk
12 × CD-ROM
33.6 kbps fax/modem

Monitor and *speakers*
Keyboard, mouse
Printer

Items in plain print are basic computer
Italics offer multimedia capability

Computer software

The program is the set of instructions that tells a computer how to manipulate digital information. Box 5.3 lists the commonest types of program.

Box 5.3. Common types of program

Operating systems (essential to make the computer work)
Word-processing
Spreadsheets
Databases
Presentation
Communication
Drawing and image manipulation
Games
Specialist tools: for instance music or video editing

These programs are given the collective term 'software'.

Operating systems

The computer operating system allows the user to interact with the computer. It files and retrieves information, presents it on the screen and controls the basic functions of the central processing unit. Early operating systems were basic and required considerable training to make them work. Modern systems present information in a *graphical user interface*, or GUI, and these systems are intuitive: you can usually get the system to work without needing handbooks or learning keyboard commands. The most important operating systems for desktop computers are:

- MS-DOS (stands for Microsoft - Disk Operating System)
- Windows (the standard Microsoft GUI produced in a variety of forms)

- Apple Systems (the first widespread GUI)
- OS-2 (a system developed for IBM by Microsoft)
- UNIX (a system widely used on business machines, and the basis of the Internet)

The operating system will determine how easy it is for you to operate your computer and therefore the speed at which you accomplish your work. Choose carefully before you buy and do not accept that this year's version of Windows is the only solution.

Having bought a computer and its associated operating system, you must then decide which of the bewildering array of programs to buy. While the basic features of a simple program can be understood within a weekend, the heavyweight commercial programs are very complex and take several months of regular use to master. It is usually sensible to buy a cheap and simple program, learn to use this, and then decide which aspects you want to upgrade. There remain several different standards for computers, check carefully to ensure that any software you buy will work with your hardware and operating system.

Word-processing

Word-processing has always been the most useful function of a personal computer. A word-processing program may be thought of as plain sheet of paper for you to write on. Word-processors enable text to be manipulated and corrected. Simple word-processors do little more than this, but more complicated programs include spelling checkers, the ability to index and to include graphics. The most complex programs allow you to create complex page layouts and are called desk-top publishing programs. Unless you plan to write and publish a book or newsletter, such complexity is unnecessary. *Word* and *WordPerfect* are common word-processors.

Spreadsheets

A spreadsheet can be thought of as an accounting book. Columns of figures can be manipulated and calculated. Trends can be analysed and graphs produced. The bigger programs interchange spreadsheet and database information and can be used to analyse data. Examples include *Excel* and *Lotus 1-2-3*.

Databases

A database is a set of electronic file cards. These store data which can be selectively extracted and analysed. Databases from several sources can be linked electronically to enable complex analyses. Basic analytical techniques are straightforward, but you need programming expertise to make use the sophisticated analysis tools of the bigger databases. Examples include *Access, Filemaker Pro* and *4th Dimension*.

Presentation programs

Presentation programs allow you to produce high quality visual aids quickly. For doctors, learning to use a presentation package should come second only to the development of word-processing skills. Examples include *Powerpoint*, *Persuasion* and *Harvard Graphics*.

Drawing and image manipulation programs

Computerized drawing programs and digitized photographs are the basis of the graphics industry and a wide range of powerful programs enable the manipulation of such digital images. Market leaders include *Corel Draw* and *Adobe Photoshop*. Any computer can handle simple images, but sophisticated image manipulation requires a powerful processor.

Communication programs

Communication programs enable one computer to link to others. Basic communications programs enable your computer to communicate with other computers via a modem or to function as a fax machine. Net-browsing software such as *Internet Explorer* and *Netscape* enables a computer to access information on the Internet.

Integrated software

Many software companies now offer suites containing relatively simple versions of each of these packages combined into a simplified whole. Such suites are a good place to start developing computer skills, examples include *Microsoft Works* or *Claris Works*. The top-end programs are also combined into suites, the best known of which is *Microsoft Office*. There are versions of these programs for each of the main operating systems.

Entertainment

Finally no one should buy a new computer without purchasing some form of educational software or game. Learning to use a computer can be dull and frustrating at times; many people will acquire the necessary skills while enjoying themselves exploring the wealth of high quality software nowadays available. Leisure software can be sub-divided into:

* *Reference works*: almanacs, dictionaries and encyclopaedias
* *Edutainments*: animated books and games aimed at teaching educational or language skills. Useful programs include those that teach one to type or use a computer more effectively
* *Adventure games*: the best are superb
* *Simulations*: fly an aircraft, run a city or rule a world. The best are excellent
* *Arcade games*: range from the addictive to the dreadful.

Computers in hospitals

Huge sums of money have been spent on attempts to computerize health care, and much of it has been wasted. Industrial computer systems running large databases for storing patient details, for payroll information or for stock-keeping, work successfully. Attempts to provide information to assist clinical staff in their work have been less successful. Thousands of hours been spent entering information into databases for management and audit, but little of this information is ever retrieved and studied.

To be successful, medical information systems must be readily accessible near to the patient and should assist rather than hinder the medical staff. Many of the problems have been technical. Over-complicated systems work slowly and staff cannot be bothered to invest the time to understand them. Clinically useful applications include:

Reporting results

Computerized reporting of investigations enables results to be distributed faster and reduces telephone calls to laboratories. Results are available to anyone in the hospital with access to the system. Tabular or graphical representations of results can be produced to assess progress of complex patients.

Order communications

Paper request forms are eliminated if clinical tests are ordered by computer. The tests can be booked in one step and ancillary staff such as radiographers, venepuncture technicians or porters co-ordinated. Doctors can be prompted by messages to ensure that they follow hospital protocols when investigating patients.

Electronic prescribing

Replacing conventional prescription cards with electronic prescribing improves the accuracy of prescribing and administrating of drugs. The system must be quick and convenient for all doctors to use. Prompts reduce the number of errors and ensure that prescriptions conform with the hospital formulary.

Electronic patient records (EPR)

Electronic patient records aim to replace the duplication, bulk, untidiness and inefficiency of the conventional paper medical record with a well-structured electronic record, which cannot become lost and which contains all relevant information. Technology has advanced to a stage where such records are feasible, but medical staff will have to change the way they work. Electronic patient records will prompt staff to undertake certain tasks — for instance remind them to measure antibiotic levels or to anti-coagulate the patient in particular clinical circumstances. Links between a hospital's clinical and financial systems will enable the cost of treatments to be calculated more efficiently.

Future developments

The dream of information enthusiasts is an EPR which integrates all hospital systems. Thus booking a patient for an elective admission to hospital would, at a keystroke, book a bed, theatre time on a particular day, organize their routine investigations, thromboembolic prophylaxis and antibiotics, and initiate the work of dieticians, physiotherapists and occupational therapists. Such information systems are theoretically possible, but may be prohibitively expensive to design and install.

Further ahead still, computers may assist medical decision making by providing clinical staff with evidence-based protocols for the treatment of both common and rare conditions. Doctors may be able to consult their colleagues and treat patients using high speed communication links and virtual reality systems. A philosophical change in the way people think is needed before such practices become commonplace.

Finally, it has been suggested that patients might carry all their medical information around with them on a credit-card sized *smart card*, which could be accessed by anyone with appropriate authority who needs to know the patient's history and therapies. Trials have been successful technically, but its benefits are unproven.

Factors hindering the development of complex information systems

Clinical staff will only accept information systems if they are:

- Easy to use
- Intuitive, and thus require minimal training
- Quick
- Efficient and effective
- Available close to the patient
- Compatible with current working practice.

Most systems installed so far do not meet these requirements, although the latest programs have a 'Windows' GUI and are much easier to use than older versions. The problem remains the high cost of electronic patient record systems. Their current cost is several million pounds for a typical district general hospital and this expense must be found from the budget available to treat patients. Once fully installed, EPRs have the potential to save considerable sums of money, both by improving the consistency of care and by reducing the risk of errors in treatment. The widespread introduction of computers into medicine has implications for the way in which doctors work and the skills they require. It is likely that many medical staff will not be able to make the necessary changes in philosophical approach.

Security

Medical records need to be seen by lots of clinicians and are insecure. Folders of notes lying around in wards or offices can be read by anyone, but access to records through computer terminals effectively multiplies the number of these records available, and allows casual access to a set of notes from any terminal without any supervision or interference from clerks or clinical staff. Medical records are sensitive, both because they contain personal information, and because there are financial implications when people try to obtain loans or buy insurance cover. Records must, therefore, be protected against casual and unauthorized access, but this is not easy. Even those authorized to access computerized records might be tempted to look at records of relatives, friends or colleagues with undesirable consequences. Once written, an electronic patient record must be tamper-proof. Most hospital information systems are now protected by personal passwords and systems that automatically disconnect a computer that has not been used for a period. When hospital computers can be accessed from outside the organization, the system should include a *firewall* that prevents unauthorized people from 'hacking' into the system and gaining access to the data stores. Sophisticated electronic record systems include 'audit trails' which record all data entries and log-ons to a particular record. Such audit trails provide greater security for information than paper-based notes.

If, for research or audit, data is downloaded to a personal computer, the data should not contain individual patient identifiers other than as a hospital or code number. An exception to this rule applies for practitioners performing private practice, who are allowed to hold details of patients on their computers for accountancy purposes. It is good practice to store the disks containing such details in a secure place separate from the computer in case the computer is stolen and the hard disk accessed. Users of personal computers may need to register under the *Data Protection Act*, but this act is concerned mainly with the collection of information for financial or marketing purposes. It would be illegal for a doctor to download a list of patients from his, or a hospital, computer if he planned to circulate them to request funds for a research project. Hospital information departments can usually supply you with information about this act.

Basic use of a computer **SKILL LEVEL 1**

Many novices are reluctant to use computers because they are afraid that their unskilled attempts damage something. In fact, modern computers are quite resistant to tampering and it is hard to inadvertently affect one unless important software is wiped. Provided that you avoid 'system folders' and 'file managers' it should be impossible for your initial attempts to create havoc. If all is not going well, save the document that you are working on, then switch the computer off for at least 20 seconds before restarting it. The computer should revert to its initial settings.

Although the graphical user interface of Windows 3, Windows 95, OS/2 and Apple operating systems differ in detail, the general principles are similar.

When the computer is switched on it performs a number of self-checks and the *desktop* then appears. The desktop consists of a top or bottom bar which contains commands, a series of illustrations (*icons*) representing the various software programs and documents on the computer hard disk and a pointer or cursor controlled by the computer mouse. Most actions on a computer can be triggered by either mouse or keyboard commands and each operating system has its own quirks. Only very general rules will be discussed in this section.

Organization of memory

Programs contain the information required to make the computer do something. A program is used to create a *document*. A document is a set of digital information which represents written, imaged or aural information. Computer memories contain many files which have to be organized so that they can be retrieved when required. Documents can be grouped into *folders*, and folders can be *nested* inside one another. The system of folders within folders is known as the *filing hierarchy*. An efficient filing hierarchy will make it easier to use your computer although the *File—Find...* command will enable you to retrieve lost documents.

The mouse

The mouse is a pointing device which has on it one or more buttons; most actions are performed using the top left button. Three actions are possible with a mouse:

- *Pointing* in which the pointer is moved to the relevant location on the screen
- *Clicking* during which the button is depressed once. Many executive actions on a computer, such as opening a program, require the button to be depressed twice in quick succession *double-clicking*
- *Dragging* in which a particular command on the menu bar is pointed at and then activated by holding the mouse button depressed. A sub-menu is revealed and moving the pointer to the sub-command while holding the button depressed triggers an action by the computer.

The menu bar

The menu bar contains the main commands controlling either the desktop or the program in current use. The most important series of commands is found by pointing and dragging on the *File* menu to the top-left of the screen. This list of commands allows one to *open, close* and *save* files as well as *print* documents. The second column of commands includes the commands *clear, copy, paste* and, very important, *undo*. Other columns of commands will vary according to the program in use.

Many programs contain a question mark icon at the top right of the menu bar. Dragging on this will usually reveal helpful information and tutorials on the use of the GUI or the program in use on the desktop. Novices should use this feature to learn about programs. In the Windows 95 operating system the menu bar may be at the base rather than the top of the screen.

Opening a program

Programs are usually stored on the computer hard disk and in most operating systems can be activated by pointing at the relevant icon and double-clicking. If using Windows '95, point at *Start* on the menu bar, click the mouse button and drag to *Program* then select the program from the menu that appears.

Saving a document

Once you have opened a program you will be presented with a blank document for you to manipulate. Soon after beginning to create something use the *File...Save as* command to store the document you have produced. You need to store this document somewhere where you can retrieve it, which maybe on a floppy disk (the *A: drive* in DOS and Windows 3) or somewhere on the hard disk (the *C: drive* in DOS and Windows 3). A floppy is easier until you have learnt how to use computerized filing systems. At regular intervals while you are working use the *File...Save* command to update this initial file. Never work for long without saving a document as a power cut or computer glitch could result in all the work you have done since the last 'save' being lost.

Closing a program

At the end of a computer session, the document in use can be put away using the *File...Close* command, and the program put away using the *File...Quit* command. If you have forgotten to save any documents these commands will prompt you to do so.

Floppy disks

The magnetic media in a floppy disk needs to be organized before the disk can be used. The disk is divided into segments and a catalogue of what is in each segment is created by *formatting* the disk. Pre-formatted disks can be purchased for IBM computers, but if you buy blank disks, or use another operating system, the computer will prompt you to format a new disk before you can save any documents onto it. Re-formatting a previously used disk destroys any information stored on it.

Printing a document

The most likely end product you require is a print-out of your work. You can see what your work looks like by using the *File...Print preview* command and, if satisfactory, you can print using *File...Print*.

Getting help

Most people learn about computers from their friends or colleagues. However, many programs now contain tutorials and help screens which can help you with specific tasks. Use the question mark command in the menu bar. The manufacturer's program manuals are often turgid and difficult to understand, but there are many informal and user-friendly instruction books available in bookshops. Buy one that suits your eyes and purse. We like the widely available ...*For Dummies* series by Greg Harvey published by Harvey IDG books. Manufacturer's telephone help lines may either help you or waste a lot of your time.

Finding out information   SKILL LEVEL 2

Knowing how to find information efficiently is becoming an essential personal skill. Obtaining and assessing medical information has become a science of its own, and is an important part of evidence-based medicine (Chapter 8). This section gives only very basic advice. If you want to know more, we recommend Trisha Greenhalgh's series of articles in the *British Medical Journal* (July–September 1997), which are gathered into *How to Read a Paper: the Basics of Evidence Based Medicine*, BMJ Publishing Group, 1997.

Medical information

Medical information can be obtained from many sources.

Books

Books are familiar and convenient. They may be accurate, but equally they can be incorrect or out-of date. There is always a delay between writing something and its appearance in print, and this can be several years for big multi-author textbooks.

Case reports

Case reports are anecdotal discussions of one, or a few cases. These can be instructive, but the reported finding may have no scientific basis.

Scientific papers

Published by journals which may peer review the content of the paper or publish it uncritically. Peer review ought to ensure that only worthwhile material is published, but depends upon the enthusiasm and knowledge of the assessor. Huge numbers of scientific papers are published each year and it is impossible for anyone to keep up-to-date with all of them except in a minute field of knowledge.

Review articles

Look at a range of papers published in a field and try to make sense of their findings. The conclusions of review articles can be affected by the way papers were selected for review and the pre-conceptions of the authors. *Systematic review articles* try to eliminate this bias by searching and analysing information scientifically rather than empirically. The value of evidence from individual papers is weighed by comparing the quality of methods used against pre-determined standards. This analysis of methodology has been termed *critical appraisal*.

Grey area information

Books, papers and reviews are usually catalogued in medical information systems. However, much that we need to know is hard to find because it is never catalogued. Unpublished research information, local and regional reports and magazine articles may affect how we think and work, but are hard to retrieve from libraries. This information is known as 'grey area literature'.

Digital information

An increasing amount of knowledge is stored digitally, either as CD-ROM or on the Internet. The advantage of digital information is that it can be searched using programs designed to pick out particular bits of information.

It is essential to recognize that any form of information is only as good as its authors. Scientific papers may be brilliant, but can also be ill-conceived, inaccurate or even fraudulent. The Internet is a valuable source of up-to-date information, but there is no control over it and something you read may be hidden advertising or the work of a crank.

Task

Select a suitable subject to investigate. The first time that you try to explore a medical topic, choose a well-demarcated subject, possibly a case or syndrome that you have to present to a ward-round, or the effects of a particular drug.

Initial information

A good general textbook remains the best starting point for your investigation. Reading it may enable you to realize what questions you should be asking. If you unsure of where to start your hunt, ask a medical librarian. The latest edition of big texts such as the *Oxford Textbook of Surgery* (or *...Medicine*) will probably include an overview of the topic and give the reference of a specialist review.

Finding out more detail

Your next step is a literature search for recent reviews and papers. Your library may have a CD-ROM database, or you may be able to use a modem linked 'on-line' system such as 'Medline'. Often these facilities have to be booked in advance. The CD-ROM database will contain the titles, references, authors and a summary of papers.

The medical librarian will show you how to use the system and advise you how to choose appropriate keywords for your search. Use of keywords in your search strategy is crucial. Too broad a search strategy will result in you finding an overwhelming amount of information, but using too limiting a set of words will mean that you miss vital information.

Transatlantic linguistic variations matter. If you are searching for information on paracetamol, you need also to enter the American name of acetaminophen, together with trade names such as Panadol and Tylenol. You must know the appropriate jargon — for instance what we call expedition medicine in the UK is known as wilderness medicine in the USA. Text modifiers such as AND and OR can help you limit your search.

Eventually you will obtain a set of papers which contain your selected keywords. Read the summaries to find which papers are relevant. Using the computer, you can select papers that you are interested in, and either store the information about them on a floppy disk or print it out.

Some of the papers you select will be available in your own library; other recent items will be accessible through the Internet and some you will have to obtain as photocopies from a central resource such as the British Library.

Looking at the internet

There are now huge amounts of information on medical subjects on the Internet. Searching the Internet requires similar strategies to searching a CD-ROM database. Use your Web browser to access one of the Internet 'search engines'. Then type in the information you want. Advanced options in the search engines allow you to specify greater detail about what you are looking for. Often you will find that you have obtained the references of a huge number of documents, and you have to try to limit your search to relevant items by adding new keywords. There is no control over information on the Internet, so the quality of information ranges from excellent to dreadful. Searching the Internet is particularly useful if you want alternative views on medical topics. For instance, if you are interested in a particular rare disease, you may find information and a discussion group run by patients suffering from this condition.

Assessing information

Once you have obtained a reasonable number of papers, you must assess their worth. Some basic factors that you might consider are listed in Box 5.4. Valuable information should be retained for future reference and the dross discarded.

Retaining information

Once you have obtained relevant information about a subject you must catalogue and store it for later use. Possibilities include keeping photocopies in

---

Box 5.4. Basic assessment of information

- How old is it?
- What type of information is it (case report/paper/review)?
- How comprehensive is it?
- Is it didactic or does it argue the topic?
- Who wrote it, and why?
- Has it been reviewed or criticized by anybody?
- Are the conclusions supported by scientific evidence?
- Does it add to your knowledge of the subject?

---

a filing cabinet, using a file card system, or maintaining a computer database of your own. Photocopies take up a lot of space, and you have to decide how to file them. It can be difficult to re-find a paper. File cards are more compact and can be coded in a variety of ways to make their information more accessible. Ensure that complete references are entered onto the card. Computer databases have many advantages. References can down be downloaded electronically from CD-ROM and on-line systems, and can be incorporated into papers. Many types of search strategy, for instance by topic, by time, or by authors, can be used to re-find information. Problems can arise when you change computers as transferring the database is not necessarily easy.

Finally

Many published papers, even in peer-reviewed journals, are flawed and you must develop a hearty scepticism of all you read. Hopefully, finding out what others have written about a subject will encourage you to explore the subject in greater detail yourself and possibly even lead to your wanting to do some research of your own in the field.

Related topics

Skill levels (pp. x–xi)
Evidence-based medicine (p. 102)

6. TALKS AND LECTURES

Objectives of this section

- to present information clearly and concisely to an audience
- to explain why some speakers are more effective than others
- to use visual aids properly
- to enable you to present a talk, research presentation or lecture

General principles

Speaking to an audience is different from writing for one. To remember what they hear, most people need to have points emphasized by visual aids and reinforced by repetition. Simple conversational speech is better than the more complex constructions of written language. The personality and presentation skills of the speaker are very important. The basic principles of lecturing are given in Box 6.1.

Box 6.1. Basic principles of lecturing

- Prepare thoroughly
- Arrive early
- Learn to work the lights
- Use prompt cards
- Speak slowly
- Stand still

- Use visual aids well
- Use gestures to emphasize
- Sense the audience
- Finish on time
- Assess your presentation

Nearly everyone feels anxious before they stand up to talk to an audience, and a degree of stress, provided that it does not lead to stage fright, helps to improve performance. Confidence comes from thorough preparation and knowledge of your material. The apparently effortless performance of a skilled lecturer is the result of many hours of preparation.

Preparation

Advance planning is essential. Consider who you will be talking to, where, for how long and what topics you will/ought to cover. A seminar for a dozen people differs from a lecture to 500. You must find out how much the audience will already know about your topic, and ensure that the contents of your talk are appropriate.

No lecture or presentation should ever run over time. A good lecturer will leave the audience wanting more, not wanting to go home! If you think you have been given too little time, either negotiate for more, or limit the scope of the talk. Do not rush through a vast range of topics as you will simply confuse the audience. Nor should you waste time saying how little time you have, or apologizing for not covering everything.

The general principles of all talks are the same:

- Tell the audience what you are going to say
- Say it and explain it
- Summarize what you have said

A first-class presentation makes the audience re-structure their ideas on a topic. You should begin by re-iterating known concepts and then add a few important bits of knowledge which will alter their understanding of the field. People like to feel reassured that they know something about a subject, but will regard the session as a waste of time if they do not come away with something new. When teaching complicated topics, prepare a handout for the audience so that they can concentrate on what you have to say, rather than spending all their time writing notes.

Arrival

Arrive well before the time for your talk, so that the chairperson is not left wondering where you are. Know the telephone number of the seminar room or conference hall so that you can make contact if you are delayed. Before your session starts, check your visual aids, the sound and lighting systems, and work out a safe way onto and off the stage. Discuss special needs with the projectionist.

Appearance

Initial impressions matter. Unless you rejoice in looking scruffy, make an effort to dress tidily, but comfortably. If your hair is long, ensure that it does not fall over your face or require constant brushing back from the eyes. As appropriate, make sure that your tie is straight, your flies zipped up, your shirt-tail tucked in and your tights ladder-free. A spare shirt or pair of tights packed in your briefcase can remedy a last minute disaster.

Speech

Look at the audience and pitch your voice as though you are holding a conversation with a person at the back of the room. Enunciate clearly and slowly, ensuring that you sound the ends of words. Begin by talking deliberately slowly, particularly if you have a national or regional accent, to allow the audience to adjust to your voice. Avoid speech mannerisms such as 'Errhh' and 'Um'. If using a static microphone, stay a fixed distance away from it; take care not to knock a portable microphone. Vary the tone of your voice so that you emphasize important points.

Body posture

Body language can make or mar your talk. Over-anxious lecturers fidget, which can be very distracting. You can disguise how you feel by sitting or standing with your feet fixed in one place. Hand and arm gestures can help to emphasize points, but use them sparingly. If you need to turn to look at a projection screen, keep your feet still and twist only your upper body. Keep your hands away from your face and hair.

A skilled lecturer scans the audience, apparently making regular eye contact with each of them. As a novice, you may find it easier simply to gaze at the middle of the audience except for the brief times when you have to point to a visual aid or glance at a prompt card. Never look at the floor and do not keep your eyes fixed on your notes. The direction of a lecturer's gaze is obvious even in a big lecture theatre. A lectern allows notes to be hidden; if using one, stand at arm's length behind it and you can then redirect your eyes from the audience to your prompt notes and back again without moving your head.

Use of notes

A skilled lecturer never appears to use a text or notes, although most will use some form of prompt.

A *full script* is a dangerous aid. The danger is that you will read aloud what you have written and that your presentation will be stilted and boring. Losing your place results in an uncomfortable delay while you re-find where you are. Some research societies forbid the use of scripts. A full script can, however, help when you are preparing a long and complex lecture. It enables you to organize your talk logically and decide how much to include. You can then learn the script for your lecture.

Prompt cards are useful. Many experienced lecturers write their introductory remarks and conclusions out in full, and then summarize the main points for each stage of the lecture on a series of postcards; often one card per projected slide. This technique gives reassurance while you are walking to the stage and provides a trigger to get you started if you are very nervous as you first face the audience. Prompt cards should be loosely fastened together with a filing (*treasury*) tag so that they can be turned easily, but cannot get out of order.

Use of visual aids

Many lecturers use slides or overhead transparencies (OHTs) to emphasize points in their talk. Chapter 7 discusses the design and production of slides and overheads. Limit the number of visual aids you use. Aim for no more than one slide per minute of lecturing up to a maximum of 60. Ideally, all the slides should have a similar design and colour scheme so that the audience can adjust to their appearance and be able to understand them more quickly. Overhead transparencies contain more information than slides and are clumsier to change. Each overhead should last for 3–4 minutes of the presentation.

Emphasize features on the visual aid by pointing; this can be done by using a torch or laser pointer directed at the screen, or by pointing the tip of a pencil at the relevant area of an OHT on the projection platter. If you are anxious, a pointer will exaggerate your tremor for all to see; be economical with your movements and use the pointer for as short a period as you can. It is usually safer to change the slides with your non-dominant hand and hold the pointer in your dominant. Some slide changers contain a laser pointer in the hand-set, but it is easy to press the wrong button and advance the slide rather than switching on the pointer. This irritates the audience and flusters the speaker.

Even experienced lecturers run into problems with visual aids and you cannot prevent projector bulbs from burning out unexpectedly. Try not to be flustered by technical problems. The lecture theatre staff should be sorting the problem out; if not, alert them to the difficulty or ask one of the organizers to fix the problem. If you are good enough, improvise until things are working again; if not, pause and wait patiently. An increasing number of lecturers use a computer-generated presentation package. Only use this technology yourself if you are confident that you can make it work.

Sensing the audience

A skilled lecturer can sense the mood of the audience and can play to it. An alert audience is quiet, with most people paying attention. Some will take notes, while others will alternate their gaze between you and your slides. A bored audience will be rustling programmes, gazing around the room, reading newspapers or talking to their neighbours and your best solution is to shorten your lecture as much as is decent. Never be upset by an elderly professor sleeping in the front row. He probably had a good lunch and is now into his normal post-prandial siesta; be flattered that he has paid you the courtesy of attending! Do not draw attention to latecomers or those who are not interested in what you have to say. You should get on with your job without getting distracted and leave them to sort themselves out.

Assessing presentations

Get into the habit of assessing talks that you attend, so that you can learn from them and improve your own presentation skills. Suitable criteria are listed in Box 6.2. Although the recommendations made in this chapter are simple and widely accepted, they are ignored by many well-known lecturers who continue to give inappropriate talks using faded slides at major conferences. They should not be invited back.

Box 6.2. Assessing a talk

- Content of talk
- Appropriateness of talk
- Clarity of ideas
- Educational value

- Use of visual aids
- Use of voice
- Body language
- Entertainment value

Presenting a clinical case   **SKILL LEVEL 1**

From the beginning of your clinical studies you have to present patient details to other doctors. Later, you have to make formal presentations to teaching or grand rounds. You should use these occasions to:

- Gain confidence in talking to an audience
- Use simple language to convey your message
- Use overhead transparencies to reinforce your verbal presentation
- Learn to answer questions effectively and succinctly

Preparation

Know about the patient. Obtain the clinical notes and work your way through them. If the notes are a mess, sort them out. Discard blank sheets of paper and put the results of investigations in order so that you know where to find data if you are asked a question during the presentation.

Write down the relevant history, findings and investigations and try to understand what has been in the minds of the clinicians at each stage. Then, if possible, talk to the patient and clarify events from their point of view. If appropriate, ask the patient's permission to use clinical photographs during the presentation. You may wish to present the patient to the round, in which case you need to explain carefully who will be there, what is going to happen and what clinical signs you want to demonstrate. Allow the patient to choose freely whether he or she wishes to participate; a grand round can be intimidating.

Visual aids

You are likely to give this presentation only once. Overhead transparencies (p. 86) are the cheapest and most appropriate way to emphasize your presentation. Use them to emphasize the sequence of events; pick out important features. A graph of laboratory results may be useful.

Typical presentation

Determine from the convenor how the meeting will be organized.

- How long should your presentation be?
- Will you be responsible for leading the discussion of the case, or will there be another chairperson?

- Should the case be presented in full initially, or in stages to discuss the development of the clinical pattern?
- Will other clinicians, for instance a radiologist or histopathologist, be involved, and if so at what stage in the presentation?

In a big lecture theatre you will need to make the presentation from a lectern, in which case ensure that you have your notes assembled and know where the pointer is. You may need an assistant to change the OHTs. In a smaller room, you can sit by the side of the OHT projector, but try to ensure that you do not shield the screen from anyone's view. Begin with demographic details — age, sex, racial origin and, if relevant, occupation.

Progress to clinical details, which are usually presented chronologically. Present only positive findings, or relevant negative findings. Clinicians tend to understand illness by a process of pattern recognition and you should give them sufficient information to accept or reject particular patterns of disease. Select relevant investigations and give these results.

Conclude by summarizing your talk, and try to stimulate discussion by listing the important issues raised by the case. Try to anticipate questions. If you know that a certain clinician often asks about a particular investigation, prepare a transparency to demonstrate the results.

In conclusion

Presenting cases is a good way to learn how to present effectively. The subject matter is well-defined, and the audience is usually small and known to the presenter. You can practise your presentation skills in a relatively benign gathering, and get immediate feedback on how well you did.

Presenting at a journal club   SKILL LEVEL 2

Journal clubs are usually informal, but if your presentation is to be worthwhile, it still requires proper preparation. You are also likely to act as the 'chair' of the meeting and this is an opportunity to learn the basic skills of controlling discussion within a group. At this stage you should concentrate on:

- Summarizing the information in a scientific paper
- Criticizing research methods and results (see also p. 107)
- Using visual aids to convey more complex information than during a case presentation
- Chairing the debate

Selecting papers

You should present either papers which deserve widespread debate, or relevant papers from journals which are not likely to have been read by the audience. It is not particularly educational to present an average paper which most people will have read anyway, unless you wish to draw attention to the methods. Always try to select articles which will provoke discussion.

You will probably be given a time-slot to fill. It is difficult to predict how long people will want to debate a particular paper, and it is unfortunate if the group does not share your enthusiasm for an article so that silence descends after a few platitudes. To avoid this problem, work through two papers in detail and become confident at presenting them, and also have a couple of 'stocking fillers', which you can present as interesting asides, but which are not likely to produce much debate. You can then mix the articles to fill the time, selecting the other long article but omitting the shorter ones if the first presentation didn't take long, or omitting the longer one and using the 'fillers' if a small amount of time is left at the end of your initial presentation. Do not overrun time yourself, although it does not matter if the debate is so heated that others decide to stay around to continue the discussion.

Visual aids

Some journal club presenters distribute photocopies of the original article to everyone attending. This breaches copyright rules, wastes paper and is a practice that should be condemned. Your aim as a presenter is to condense the information and point out the bits that matter. Another poor technique is to photocopy a page from the journal directly onto an OHT. The text that appears on the OHT will be far too small for most people to read and, even if highlighted, is not an effective way of emphasizing information. Instead cut out the important text and graphics from a first-generation photocopy of the article, paste them onto a new sheet and enlarge them on a photocopier. These abbreviated sheets can then be used as the basis for your OHT, or as part of a short handout if the presentation is to take place at a home.

Debate

Begin your presentation by saying what prompted you to present the article and why you think that it is interesting. The published results may be interesting in their own right, but the point of debating the paper should be to determine whether the meeting thinks that:

- The methods were satisfactory
- The statistics were applied correctly
- The conclusions were reached appropriately
- The results are applicable to clinical or research practice

You should structure your presentation with these points in mind and make sure that you have relevant knowledge to answer questions. If you are not a statistician, try to look up the tests that were used and see if they seem appropriate. If you think them inappropriate, discuss them with an expert. At the end of your presentation, make clear what points you think should be debated and then make it clear that the debate should start. You may then need to revert to a chairman's role.

Chairing debates

When leading a discussion it is important to maintain control. Try to ensure that only one person talks at a time. Signal clearly who has the floor and try to discourage others from talking simultaneously. If several people are keen to contribute, suggest that Dr A should speak next, followed by Drs B and C. This usually keeps people under control. Allow follow-up remarks to a statement before going on to the next speaker if the remarks were especially contentious. If someone leads the discussion astray, guide it back to the original subject. Keep an eye on the clock and draw the discussion to a firm conclusion as the proportion of valuable comments declines. Try to summarize the conclusions of the debate.

Research presentations   SKILL LEVEL 3

If you become involved in research you will have to present your findings. Venues for research presentations range from your own hospital to national or international forums. All settings can be equally nerve-wracking. The approach you take to presenting research work should be the same for all types of meeting, although you may wish to modify your presentation to suit a particular audience. Depending on the progress of your research you may be presenting: an ongoing study, an abstract of pilot data, or completed work. The skills you require are:

- Writing and submitting a research abstract for a meeting
- Conveying scientific information clearly
- Keeping precisely to time
- Minimizing reliance on notes during the presentation
- Producing and using slides effectively (p. 87)
- Preparing for questions from the floor

Applying to present your research

Senior academic staff will expect you to submit your research for discussion at an appropriate meeting. Choose a meeting at which you will be able to discuss your findings with other workers in the same field. It is very desirable if your supervisor or friends can also attend the meeting to give you moral support.

Obtain an application form from the meeting organizers. You will usually be required to submit an abstract 3–6 months ahead of the date of the meeting. This will be reviewed and you will be informed of the reviewer's decision. You may be able to choose whether you want to present your data as a poster or as a talk, but this decision may be made for you.

The application forms for a society meeting usually have very specific instructions about the length of the abstract and the appearance of diagrams or tables. Some are now available on computer disk, but if you are sent a form, you should make several photocopies of the application sheet and use these for the drafts as inevitably you will make initial mistakes. If you look at published abstracts from previous meetings of the relevant society you will see how researchers use different fonts and spacing to shrink or enlarge their work appropriately.

Start by typing your abstract on a word-processor, you can then use different font sizes and line spacing so that it fits the appropriate area. Alternatively you can use a photocopier to shrink or enlarge text and diagrams and then paste these onto the application form. Finally photocopy the whole document so that it looks neat and professional. Remember that some department secretaries are familiar with typing abstracts to fit application forms and they may be able to save you a lot of time and effort.

Planning

When your work is accepted for presentation be sure you are clear about the date, time and venue for the presentation and the form it will take. Presentations are of two types: the poster presentation and the verbal presentation. Begin the preparation of slides or posters well in advance. Think about funding for travel, hotel expenses and the meeting fee. Registration fees are usually reduced or omitted for presenters.

Poster presentations

This is the easier and less stressful form of presentation. You should be sent guidelines for the dimensions of the display area. If you have not prepared a poster before go to the medical illustration department in your hospital and ask to see some examples. You will then get ideas about how to present your data and find out how the department can help you. Ask how long it takes to lay-up and laminate your material onto the poster board. Standards of presentation vary widely but you should aim to produce a poster that looks good as well as demonstrates good quality research.

The information you display can be based on your submitted abstract but you may have more data to add and you will certainly have more room for explanatory text and figures. You should include subsections such as the method, the results and a discussion, together with a summary.

You should be sent information about when and where to display your poster, as well as being told the times at which you are required to stand by it to answer questions from interested colleagues. If you do not receive these details well in advance, contact the conference secretariat to get them to send you details. Remember to take appropriate references and information with you as it is likely that you will be questioned in depth about your work. This is less like a viva and more like a friendly chat between enthusiasts and you should look upon it as a chance for swapping ideas.

Other points to consider:

- If you are travelling abroad consider making your poster as a laminated sheet that can be rolled up
- Traditional hardboard posters can be made in sections that are easy to carry
- Do not pack the poster in your suitcase as luggage can get lost

Remember to take a supply of adhesive tape, drawing pins and scissors for running repairs.

Verbal research presentations

Verbal research presentations can be extremely intimidating. It may be the first time you have stood up in front of a large audience, and you may be faced by people who enjoy picking holes in other's research work. Remember that you and your co-workers will know more about your research than anyone else. You must present your information clearly, starting from basics. Plan to talk for slightly less than the allotted time. Your pace will probably be slower than your practice speed and you need to allow time for questions.

When you start to prepare your presentation write it out in full, using as a guide the format of most publications — introduction (including why *you* did the work), method, results, discussion. But, remember to personalize it. Keep slides easy to read and understand. It may be appropriate to use video clips to illustrate your work, but check that video equipment will be available at the meeting.

Practise your presentation so that you can present it without referring to notes or crib sheets, although having them there for comfort or a moment of panic is sensible. It is worthwhile trying out your presentation on members of your department, particularly those who are familiar with research presentations. Do this sufficiently far ahead of the meeting that the talk can be revamped or slides changed if appropriate. You need to get feedback on your style of presentation (clarity of speech and body language) as well as scientific content. The questions that your colleagues ask may give a clue to what you will be asked at the meeting and this will enable you to prepare answers. Consider making back-up slides to clarify these replies. Label and number all slides clearly in case you drop them while putting them in the projector cassette.

Before you go to the meeting read around the subject again; it may even be worth repeating a literature search to ensure that you are aware of the latest publications on your subject. Take the relevant references with you.

Plan to get a good night's sleep the night before your presentation; avoid the local hostelries and boisterous colleagues. Dress sensibly. Present yourself to the meeting moderator who should instruct you about slide or video projection. Check that your slides are in order and run through them to see that they are all the correct way up. When your turn comes try some deep slow breathing exercises and then speak slowly and clearly. Good luck!

Lecturing SKILL LEVEL 4

In other skill sections in this chapter, you have had to transmit a limited amount of well-structured information to your audience. As you become more senior you are likely to be invited to lecture to students or colleagues within your department or at a conference or society. When you lecture you should aim to be a teacher and entertainer as well as simply a presenter. The basic rules are those already described but in addition you should try to:

- Prepare an effective summary of a complex topic
- Convey the key points in this summary to others
- Present your lecture in an entertaining and dynamic fashion

Initial contacts
You will usually be contacted by phone or letter by the conference or course organizer or society secretary. Discuss with the organizer exactly what is required. Agree a length for your slot and find out if you have to leave time for questions. Find out who the audience will be and what they will expect of you. If other lecturers are going to talk on related topics, find out how to contact them so that you do not cover the same ground. If you intend to charge a fee or will need accommodation discuss your requirements now so that there are no embarrassing misunderstandings. A good organizer will confirm the arrangements in writing.

Preparing a lecture
Lectures require a lot of preparation; a minimum of 10 hours preparation for a 1 hour lecture. The lecturers with the most informal style are usually those who have spent the greatest time preparing their talks. Think about the subject that you have to talk about. Read around the topic in detail several weeks before you are expected to give the lecture. Then leave the books alone for a period and see what you remember as the most important aspects.

What are the messages that you want to convey? Write them down and use them as the skeleton for the talk. In a lecture, you need not, and generally should not, describe detailed research techniques and findings. Instead, paint a picture for the audience of the subject, summarizing the evidence for your statements in a couple of effective slides. Once you know what you want to say, prepare the script of your lecture in detail. Unless you are an expert with a good sense of timing, avoid jokes, which are likely to fall flat, and cynical remarks which may irritate some sections of the audience. Slides are for reinforcing the main points of the talk and should be prepared only after you know what you are going to say. When everything is prepared, rehearse the talk with colleagues and listen to their comments. Make sure your lecture is shorter than the time allocated to you. Learn it well.

Just before the talk

Contact the organizer again to finalize travel arrangements and timing. If you need dual projection, video or an X-ray box make sure that they will be available. Lecture halls usually have OHT and slide projectors, but other venues may not and you may have to take your own.

On arrival

Make yourself known to the organizers as soon as you arrive; it will stop them worrying. Check your slides in the projector. Discover how the slide changer and light dimmers work. Microphones can be a menace; discover where to clip a lightweight microphone or how close you need to be to a static microphone. Discuss your requirements with the projectionist. Avoid over-indulgence if a meal precedes the talk. It is a grave discourtesy to your audience to ignore these preparations.

On stage

Make use of all your skills. Put on the microphone if you need it. Start speaking slowly so that the audience get used to your voice. Enunciate clearly. Make eye contact with your audience and scan across them. Do not turn your body to face the slides or mumble at the lectern. Keep your feet still. Avoid repetitive habits, such as sweeping hair back from your eyes or scratching your nose. Arm gestures can be valuable if not overdone. Use the pointer sparingly. Do not overstay your welcome.

Things that go wrong

Your advance preparation should have reduced the risk of disasters. You should know how to control the sound and lighting systems but, if you get stuck, ask the chairperson to sort out your problem. A spare set of OHTs, which include the most important points of the lecture, can help out if you lose your slides or there is an irremediable projector fault such as a blown bulb with no spare. Acoustics are always a problem; dispense with the microphone altogether if the sound system is dreadful and you have the ability to project your voice adequately. If you have to give a lecture abroad, try to discover the main language of the audience and the arrangements for translation. Simultaneous translation will allow you to get more information across in the allotted time than if you have to pause to allow time for translation.

Question time

The stupidest person can ask a question that the cleverest person cannot answer so do not be fazed by this; however, some people try to score points off you to show how clever they themselves are. Such bores can be dealt with firmly, though politely. Answer even the most stupid question politely; it may have been your fault the questioner did not understand in the first place.

Afterwards

You will have had some idea about how well your talk was received by observing what proportion of the audience were concentrating on what you were saying. Ask the organizer to send on the results of the course assessment form. Finally, keep your notes and slides well organized in case you are asked back to repeat the talk.

Related topics

Visual aids (p. 81)
Chairing a group (p. 126)

7. VISUAL AIDS

Objectives of this section
- to understand the benefits and drawbacks of different media
- to be able to design an effective and legible visual aid
- to use a computer program to produce a visual aid

You do not need visual aids to give a lecture. Many great speakers use none. However, if you are seeking to communicate complex scientific information, aids can:

- Give obvious structure to your talk or lecture
- Form a basis for your audience to make notes
- Summarize complex information as pictures or graphs.

Visual aids make or mar a lecture. Computers enable anyone to create smart and effective professional standard graphics quickly, but too often one sees slides in which style outweighs content and inappropriate use of colour reduces information to invisibility.

The media

Blackboards and whiteboards

Drawing boards are ideal for jotting down thoughts or explaining ideas during informal tutorial groups. You can develop ideas as you talk, allowing the audience to see how you construct an equation, graph or result. The end product is ephemeral and usually untidy, so these aids should not be used for formal presentations, or in big lecture theatres.

Dusty chalk boards have been largely replaced by whiteboards. When using a whiteboard, make sure to use the correct type of pen. Permanent markers cannot be erased and damage whiteboards. The correct pens can be erased with a dry rubber, but the whiteboard needs to be cleaned at intervals with water or an appropriate solvent. Before you begin your presentation, ensure that the pens still work. Write large, legibly and preferably horizontally. Cap the pens between uses. Use the correct side of the board rubber; its working surface will cover you and your clothes with coloured dust.

Flipboards

Many seminar rooms are now equipped with paper flipboards. These pads of cheap paper are beloved of management consultants, but are really no more than a small, less ecologically sound whiteboard. Their advantage is that some sheets can be produced before the start of the seminar, thus saving time during the talk. Discussions can be summarized by flipping over the pages.

Overhead projectors

Most lecture theatres and seminar rooms are equipped with overhead projectors. They are an effective way of demonstrating information to small or large audiences. Before using an overhead projector, make sure that you know how to switch it on and off, that the projection platter is dirt-free, and that the lens is dust-free and correctly focused. Position the projector carefully. If it is too close or too far below the screen, the illuminated square becomes severely distorted with coloured fringes. The edges of the projection area are often out of focus so you should use a 20 cm square format for your OHTs, although you can use a longer vertical height if you plan to uncover your OHT in sequence and do not wish to retain all the field in view. If you are giving your talk from near the projector, make sure that you do not obscure parts of the screen from the audience.

Overhead transparencies can be handwritten using washable or permanent fibre-tips. Writing film 'acetates' are cheap and reusable, making them ideal for use at once-only informal meetings such as case presentations. However, it is difficult to write neatly and a smarter solution for formal presentations is to word-process the text (see pp. 86–87) and then print the result either from paper onto OHT film using a photocopier, or print directly onto special transparency film using an inkjet or laser printer. Mounts can be bought for OHTs that you re-use regularly and these allow you to superimpose films to build up a complex picture.

Very important: The OHT film used in laser printers and photocopiers differs from the film that you write on and is much more expensive (about 30p per sheet). Use photocopying OHTs sparingly and never put ordinary acetates into a laser printer or photocopier — it will melt and cause expensive damage to the copying drum. Special OHT film is also made for colour inkjet printers; this costs about 45p per sheet. The only certain way to differentiate the various types of film is to read the package label.

Slides

For many years 35 mm slides have been the most popular medium for transmitting visual information. The recent development of computerized presentation programs has made it easier and quicker to produce effective slides. Most hospital doctors have to give lectures and should be able to design their own slides (see pp. 87–90). It is worthwhile building up a library of slides relevant to your work. Slides can be used many times, but you must store them in a dark dry place to minimize the rate at which they deteriorate. A colour slide costs at least 50p to produce, and a commercial agency may charge you five to ten times this amount.

The quality of projection facilities in lecture theatres varies widely. You should design slides that remain legible even if the theatre has inadequate blackout facilities or bright auditorium lights. Design slides in horizontal 'landscape' format, rather than vertical format, as projection screens are often too short to allow all of a vertical slide to be projected.

Dual projection

Some lecturers try to increase the impact of their presentation by using two slide projectors to produce a wide-screen effect. Few manage to use the technique successfully. It works well in two circumstances:

1. A single summary slide is projected onto one side of the screen while the rest of the slides are projected onto the other half of the screen.
2. One projector is used for photographs or graphics while the other projector is used for text. Each projector has an equal number of slides and each pair is changed together.

Any attempt to advance each side separately is liable to end in chaos, unless you use a pre-programmed automatic slide-changer. Dual projection should never be used simply to cram more information into a lecture.

Videos

Large lecture theatres will have facilities to project videos. Drug or equipment manufacturers often produce videos to promote their wares, and because they can include interviews and moving graphics they are a useful teaching medium. Unfortunately, we are all used to the high standards of television presentation and it is hard for amateurs to match these. Probably for this reason, personally produced videos are rarely used by medical lecturers, though there is no reason why someone with a particular interest and expertise in this medium should not use them.

Computer-generated presentation packages

An increasing number of lecture theatres have a computer and video projector. These allow a lecturer to project graphics, produced using a presentation program, directly from a computer disk onto screen. Photographs, sound, video clips and numerous visual effects can be incorporated into the presentation; but remember that simplicity is a virtue and resist the temptation to use too many special effects. An expert can produce or modify a slide very quickly. Digital disks can be duplicated easily and are portable, thus reducing the risk of losing, damaging or dropping a box of slides during travel. Although the purchase cost of the equipment is high, the only production cost for the graphics is the 50p of the floppy disk on which the data is stored.

If you plan to use your own computer, make sure that you have the correct video connections with you to link the computer to the projector, and beware of the 'sleep' system built into many laptops, which can shut the computer down unexpectedly if no keystrokes are made for a period. If using the lecture theatre's computer system, make sure that their computer has software compatible with the program that you used to produce the slides.

Graphic design

Visual aids should be simple, clear and uncluttered. When you start, design your slides so that they contain no more than 24 words, 16 items of information or one graph. Use all the available space.

General appearance

Although the 'Windows' and 'Mac' computer screens are supposed to be 'WYSIWYG', which means 'what you see is what you get', this is only approximately true. Monitor definition is only 72 points per inch, while a good printer will smooth appearances to 600 dpi. Some lettering will print-out differently from the way it appears on screen, while colours on the screen rarely match the final printed or slide version.

Lettering

The appearance of a typeface is described as its *font* (Box 7.1). Fonts may have twiddly bits and are described as *serif*, or have a plainer appearance and be *sans-serif*. Text is usually written in a serif font, while headings and notices are usually sans-serif. The letters of the font may be equally spaced in the manner of a typewriter, or may be a variable space apart to produce a more integrated appearance. This is known as *proportional spacing* and most computer fonts are proportionately spaced. In most word-processing packages the *spacing* between the letters and lines can be adjusted and the size of the print varied. Normally 10 *point* or 12 point font *size* is used for writing letters, but larger sizes are needed for graphics. The text itself can be enhanced by underlining it, making it bold or using italics. Avoid mixing fonts on one slide.

Box 7.1. Typefaces

Arial and **Helvetica** are sans-serif fonts
Times New Roman is a serif font, with more 'twiddly bits'
All these fonts are proportionately spaced, but `Courier`
`is a fixed space font`
Bold, *Italic* and <u>underlining</u> can usually be specified
using the menu bar

This is 16 point Times New Roman in comparison to the normal 12 point

Variation in spacing can alter appearance, but this is still Times New Roman

---

Alignment

The text can be *aligned* to one or other margin, or *centred* about the midline. It can also be *justified,* which means that the spaces between words are adjusted to ensure that both margins are aligned down the page. Headings are usually centred, but it is easier to read text aligned to the left margin than centred scripts.

Colour

Colour reproduction involves complex technology. Graphics that look smart on a computer screen often reproduce inaccurately on an OHT or slide, and the end-result is illegible. Avoid juxtaposing deep, dark, that is *heavily saturated* colours, as there will be little contrast between them, and text will be difficult to read. Instead contrast pale pastel colours with strong ones. Choose a dark background for slides such as royal blue, maroon or a strong green as slides with these colour schemes do not show dust and dirt. Add script or graphs in white, pastel yellow, orange or pale blue. Although combinations of deep red and deep blue look nice on a computer monitor, do not combine them. The eye focuses red and blue light differently and slides containing both are always hard to read.

Displaying data

Tables and graphs should be simple, so that the audience can understand unfamiliar data quickly. A visual aid that needs extensive explanation is badly designed. Simple information such as demographic data, or one column of figures, is best presented as a table. If two small data series are to be compared, a table usually remains the best choice. If you would end up with more than three columns and four rows on your chart, the slide will be difficult to read and you should consider presenting the information as a graph instead.

Designing graphs

It is the information contained in the graph that matters, not the elegance of the graphics. The basic elements of any graph are:

- The title
- Labelled axes
- Clearly marked scales, but not too many grid points
- The plot
- Error bars if it is a scientific plot
- The legend if several data series are plotted

Think what you are plotting and choose the appropriate type of display. If you are illustrating proportions, use a pie diagram. Discrete points should be plotted on an *x/y* plot, while values should be displayed as a histogram. Aim for simplicity, the best graphs are those in which all extraneous information is excluded and the message is immediately obvious. Make use of all the available space on the slide.

Modern presentation programs contain many features to 'enhance' your graphics. These include the ability to add three dimensions, vary the scales, add numerous colours and tilt the whole illustration. These features are tempting, but ask yourself very carefully whether they will allow you to convey any additional information. Occasionally they will have genuine benefits; more often they add style but no substance and you should avoid them. Most of these enhancements are designed to allow graphic designers and advertisers to manipulate data. Graphs are often manipulated to influence the reader; common tricks are listed in Box 7.2.

Box 7.2. Inappropriate graphical design

- Tilting graphs to produce false alignments between scale and data
- Using scales with a common origin, but not including the zero
- Magnifying changes by markedly expanding scales
- Using non-linear scales inappropriately
- Making interpretation impossible by drawing 'exploded' graphs which lack true axes
- Altering the size of pie diagrams without explanation

Assessing visual display of data

In Box 6.2, (p. 71) we suggested ways of assessing presentation skills. Box 7.3 suggests how you can judge a speaker's use of visual aids.

Box 7.3. Assessment of the quality of visual aids

- Does the speaker obscure the screen from the audience?
- Can the speaker control the projectors, lights and microphones?
- Are visual aids in the correct order, correctly oriented and clean?
- Are the slides or OHTs legible and uncluttered, with no unnecessary adornments?
- Do the slides need to be explained before they can be understood?
- Is all the projected text clearly visible at the back of the room?
- Does the speaker use the pointer sparingly and effectively?

Producing a basic OHT · SKILL LEVEL 2

These instructions teach you how to produce a simple OHT using a computer word-processing package. The production of transparencies using a cut-and-paste technique is discussed in the section on presenting at a journal club (p. 72). It is assumed that you have basic computer skills (p. 60).

1. Open your word-processing package. A4 is the usual default page size. Alter the **margins** so that your page set-up is 7 inches or 18 cm square, this means that the margins are about 1.5 cm or 0.7 inch from the horizontal page edge and 5 cm or 2 inches from top and bottom. In most programs margins are altered using the *File—Page Setup...* command.

2. **Type** your heading. Press the *return* key twice, then carry on by typing each line of your text and then pressing the *return* key. Minimize the number of words you use, ideally no more than one line per sub-heading in the finished form. Divide text into easily visible blocks by returning twice at the end of each group of topics; otherwise use the return key at the end of each sentence. The simplest way to indent text is to use the tab key, although more experienced users will vary the margin position.

3. When all the text is typed, you need to format it. First select the **heading** by *dragging* the mouse cursor over it. Change it to a sans-serif font such as Arial or Helvetica. Embolden the heading, but do not underline it. The *font size* should be at least 28 pt. *Centre* it. These changes can usually be performed using the mouse and clicking on the appropriate buttons in the formatting bar at the top of the screen, but can also be achieved using the *Format—Font...* and *Format—Alignment...* commands.

4. Next select all the **text** and apply Arial or Helvetica at 16 pt or above. If the text looks crowded increase the spacing between lines to 1.5 or double using the *Format—Paragraph...* command. Emphasize parts of the text by selectively bolding words or applying 'bullet marks'. Selecting paragraphs and then using the *Format—Borders...* command will allow you to draw boxes around parts of the text, but avoid shading as it will not reproduce well when projected. Italics are occasionally useful.

5. **Print** the finished page using a good quality printer. Now obtain a sheet of OHT copier film, which usually consists of the clear layer of film and a paper backing. Your paper print-out is placed on the photocopier platter in the usual way and the OHT film is fed, transparent side UP, through the single sheet feeder of the photocopier. Keep multiple films separated by their paper dividers as they can otherwise stick together and transfer printing.

6. Label the OHTs so that you know what order they should be in.

Using a presentation program   SKILL LEVEL 3

This section gives brief instructions on producing slides or overheads using a typical presentation program, and should enable you to produce visual aids for your first slide presentation. This explanation assumes that you possess basic computer skills (p. 60). Details of formatting commands apply to Microsoft™ Powerpoint, although most presentation programs use similar commands.

Before you start

Re-read the advice on graphic design given earlier in this section. Slides must be simple and uncluttered. When you first use a presentation program it is easier to design the slides as paper sketches rather than trying to compose them while simultaneously learning a new computer program.

The *Help* facility in the program offers tutorials as well as instruction on how to complete particular tasks if you get stuck.

Initial stage

- Open the presentation program in the usual way
- The initial window will ask you to select a format for your presentation. Select *Blank presentation* and click OK
- You will then be offered a series of slide types. Choose *Title slide*, click OK and a blank slide will appear
- Click in the top box and type the title of your talk. Select the whole script by dragging across it. Choose a font you like from the list given in the font selector on the formatting menu bar. Times, Times New Roman, Arial or Helvetica are safe options. Then click the **B** and the **S** buttons. This will make your script stand out by making it bold and *shadowing* the text. The default *font size* of 44 point is usually adequate, although you may sometimes choose to use a larger script
- Next click on the lower 'sub-title' box on the slide and repeat the process for your name, co-workers and department. Use a smaller font size and avoid the bold and shadow enhancements as you will then emphasize the difference between the two parts of the slide. Now *save* your work to a computer disk, noting where the file is stored

Slide production

Now work through your slides. For each new slide, click *New slide* on the bottom bar. You can move forwards or backwards through your stack of slides using the double arrowhead buttons on the vertical bar to the right of the composition window.

- Choose an appropriate slide layout each time. 'Bulleted lists' or 'two column lists', are the most useful options
- If you use the default font sizes, you will be safe. Do not shrink text below 26 point as it will not be easy to read
- The emphasis points, or bullet marks, can be removed by selecting lines of script and clicking on the bullet button towards the right hand end of the menu bar
- As far as possible use the tab key to align text rather than the space bar
- If your slide layout includes a heading and subtext, bold and shadow the heading as you did for the title slide
- Graphs, flow charts and pictures can all be incorporated, but you are recommended to seek expert advice the first time you try this

- Every five slides or so, save your work again. Continue until you have produced all your slides

Formatting

- Before formatting the presentation, make sure that you have saved all your work to computer disk in case you make a mistake at this stage
- Check the spelling of your slides both by reading them very carefully and by using the *Tools—Spelling...* command. Make sure you have used capital letters consistently
- If you plan to use OHTs, you can now simply print them out onto A4 size paper. Go to the *File—Slide set-up... Slides sized for...* pick list and select the *A4 paper* box. Then go to *File—Print* and produce your text onto paper. You can then photocopy the material onto overhead transparencies
- More work needs to be done if you plan to get slides produced or use computer graphics. Initially go to *File—Slide set-up...* and select *35 mm slide* from the *Slides sized for...* pick list
- Next format the background by going to: *Format—Slide background....* When the appropriate window opens, select *Change color...* and a safe option is to choose a strongly saturated royal or navy blue. You can vary the darkness of this using the slide bar in the window. Many people shade their slides and sometimes it improves the appearance. Initially only shade 'vertically' and choose the option with the paler colour at the top and darker at the bottom. This option is used because many big lecture theatres have overhead lights which shine onto the bottom of the projection screen and make contrast worse low down. Click *OK*
- Your dark text may now be barely visible, but this is easily sorted out by going back into *Format—Slide color scheme*. Click on the box labelled *Title text* followed by *Change color*. Choose yellow. Repeat the process for *Text and lines* and choose white. When you have completed this task, click *OK*, return to your slides and see what you have produced. You can play around a bit by changing the format and colour of the bullet marks, but you should have produced a reasonably clear and simple set of slides

To look at your slides use the slider on the right hand side of the screen to move to slide 1 and then click on the *Slide viewer* button at the bottom of the screen. You will see your slides in all their glory. View them from 10 ft foot away in a well-lit room. They should be easy to read. If they are difficult to read, no one in the lecture theatre will be able to understand them and you need to redesign them.

You may later decide to explore the possibilities that the pre-designed templates, clipart and other features that presentation programs offer, but you are unlikely to make clearer slides than when you use these simple designs.

Save all your work to a floppy disk and make a copy in case one is lost. You can either take this with you if the lecture hall has computer graphics projection facilities, or you can give it to your medical illustration department to produce your slides. You need to make sure that your version of the presentation program is compatible with the one that your department uses, seek advice if you need to transfer a file between different versions of Windows or between a Macintosh computer and a PC.

Further reading

Doig Simmonds and Linda Reynolds, *Data Presentation and Visual Literacy in Medicine and Science*. Butterworth Heinemann, Oxford, 1994.
A compact paperback which contains valuable additional hints on page and poster design and layout.

Edward R Tufte, *The Visual Display of Quantitative Information*. Graphics Press, Box 430, Cheshire, CT 06410, USA, 1983.
A beautiful and fascinating book for those interested in graphical design.

Related topics

Small group teaching (p. 41)
Computers and information technology (pp. 51–66)
Talks and lectures (pp. 67–79)

8. QUALITY IN MEDICINE

Objectives of this section

- to understand what is meant by 'quality'
- to define: audit, evidence-based medicine, quality assurance and risk management
- to collect data and complete a clinical audit project
- to consider whether these techniques change doctors' clinical practice

In mediaeval times medicine was little more than a combination of witch-craft and quackery. Nowadays, doctors receive a scientific training and should use contemporary knowledge to select the best treatments for their patients. As medicine has moved from an art to a science, and as it has consumed a greater proportion of nations' wealth, politicians and society have demanded that doctors become more accountable. Clinical audit, risk management and evidence-based medicine are mechanisms that have been established to try to ensure that resources are used properly and treatment is effective. They have been introduced so that the 'quality' of health care improves, but this commonly-used word must be defined.

Quality

Quality is a hard word to define; its dictionary definition is *degree of excellence*. The deliberately ambiguous definition: *Quality is what you like* appeals to cynics. Neither definition improves our understanding of quality in health care. There are three practical definitions of quality care that are worth considering:

1. *Care of the type that you would yourself like to receive.* This definition has certain merits, but can be criticized for suggesting that the aspirations of predominantly male Anglo-Saxon senior hospital consultants match those of the population in general. Reforms of obstetric care and changes in the management of AIDS patients took place because client/patient groups had wishes different from the care offered by providers.

2. *The most cost-effective care available.* This definition can be criticized because there are always some managers who seek to restrain costs more than others. In health care there is rarely any obvious link between cost and results.

3. Modern consumer organizations should be 'customer-centred' and the concept that *a quality organization is one that meets the expectations of its*

customers has much to commend it. Application of this concept in a market economy explains a lot of apparent anomalies in consumer surveys. For instance, most observers regard the absolute quality of a Mercedes car to be greater than that of a Skoda. However, the expectations of a Mercedes owner are rather higher than those of a Skoda owner and this explains why consumer surveys regularly show that Skoda owners are more satisfied overall with their purchase that those of the more expensive German marque. Similarly the expectations of a private patient may be greater than those of an NHS patient and they may regard the care offered as of lower quality unless special efforts are made.

Doctors can now offer far more sophisticated health care than most countries can afford. Patients' expectations have increased faster than the health-care systems' ability to meet them. As a result, people believe that the quality of care is falling. The dilemma in health care is that most patients have few comparative experiences on which to judge their care. The aim of the *Patient's Charter* was to suggest the minimum national standards that they should expect.

Cost is not the only consideration in health care. Discussions of quality must consider *equity, humanity* and *clinical effectiveness*. Doctors accept that clinical effectiveness is desirable. Equity and humanity are moral issues and provoke argument. Some people are more equal than others, and assertive individuals will often be able to use the system more effectively than those less knowledgeable about health care. Money will buy earlier treatment in nicer surroundings, whether it should depends upon your point of view.

Quality circles

The desire to provide good medical care has led to an understanding that its quality should be judged by explicit, consistent and measurable standards. Such standards should be monitored regularly and attempts continually made to improve on the existing position. This concept is the basis of the *quality circle* (Box 8.1), a management technique first used by Japanese industry in the post-war years. Quality circles can be used to analyse clinical, educational or management processes.

All hospitals routinely collect large amounts of data. To be helpful in decision making, these data must be analysed and turned into meaningful information. This new knowledge, combined with previous information and experience, can then be used to alter the way things are done and, hopefully, improve care. Change should be monitored against explicit indicators, standards and targets.

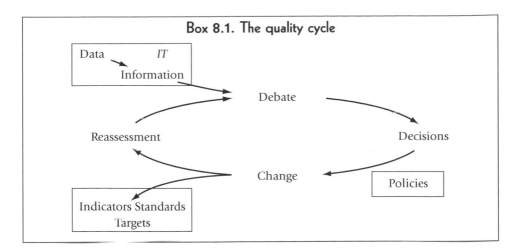

Box 8.1. The quality cycle

Standards
The minimum level of care which it is expected that an individual or organization will provide. Remedial action must be taken if the quality of care falls below this level. There are only a few clinical situations which permit the use of compulsory standards, but examples include the expectation that patients will be properly identified before undergoing a surgical procedure, and that there will be a swab count at the end of the operation.

Indicators
Measures of how effectively an organization is performing. The best known indicator is the hospital waiting list, but British hospitals have to provide government with a huge range of information from waiting times in out-patients to the efficiency of their heating systems.

Targets
Indicator levels which the organization seeks to achieve. The *Health of the Nation* has set many targets for improving the overall health of the population. Examples include: that breast cancer deaths in the population of women invited for screening should be reduced by 25% in 2000 compared to 1990, and that by 2005 the proportion of obese adults should be 7% or less.

Bringing about change
It is immensely difficult for a big organization to alter the way that things are done. Even a simple change will have far-reaching consequences. In theory 'quality-management techniques' permit the introduction of logical and sensible improvements in care. In practice the difficult bit is to get people to agree to anything! The key principles of using quality circle as a method of changing the way health is delivered are listed in Box 8.2. Although logical, many factors external to the debate impede efforts to produce change; lack of money being the most obvious. The perpetual diffi-

> ## Box 8.2. Using quality circles to produce change
>
> - Everyone in the organization should be involved more or less equally
> - Debate is based upon knowledge both of 'best practice' and of the prevailing local situation
> - Debate results in the development of explicit standards of practice
> - Everyone should be either prepared to co-operate or be coerced into accepting them
> - Indicators should be developed which can be used regularly to assess whether practice is moving towards the desired targets
> - That having achieved the initial target, the topic should be debated again to seek further improvements in practice

culty of producing real change is the reason why many doctors have become disillusioned by the audit process.

Clinical audit

Audit is defined as: *the systematic and critical analysis of the quality of clinical care, including the procedures used for diagnosis, treatment and care, the associated use of resources and the resulting outcome and quality of life for the patient.*

Audit versus research

Medical research seeks universal truths which are applicable to patients everywhere, while clinical audit is primarily concerned with ensuring that the care offered locally by individuals, departments or hospitals is as effective as possible. Research should always precede audit so that decisions can be made on the basis of best practice. Such research should be balanced and comprehensive, hence the development of *evidence-based medicine*. Retrospective research studies have often been called audit, but are nowadays considered to be 'pre-audit' as the audit process is concerned with the setting and monitoring of explicit standards. Morbidity and mortality discussions are usually regarded as *quality assurance* rather than audit.

Development of clinical audit

Audit is not a new idea (Box 8.3) and medical audit has flourished in Britain for 50 years. The balance between confidentiality and accessibility of information differs between Britain and North America, and this has made it easier for the British to undertake long-term studies such as the Maternal Mortality and Peri-operative Deaths audits. Doctors have been prepared to discuss their management of cases assured that the information will remain anonymous. Valuable lessons have been learned.

Box 8.3. Development of audit

1904　Hey Groves recommends standardization of operation names

1924　US College of Surgeons begins to accredit hospitals

1952　UK sets up Confidential Enquiry into Maternal Deaths

1956　Association of Anaesthetists Enquiry into Operative Deaths

1987　Confidential Enquiry into Peri-operative Deaths (CEPOD)
　　　 studies the anaesthetic and surgical professions in Britain

1989　British government White Paper funds increased audit activity in
　　　 the National Health Service

1994　Official move from funding uniprofessional medical audit to
　　　 multi-disciplinary clinical audit.

At the time of the re-organization of the NHS consequent upon the 1989 White Paper, there were few areas of agreement between the government and the doctors representing the medical profession. The idea that audit was worthwhile was one area of common ground and, possibly as an appeasement measure, funding was made available to introduce medical audit as a regular feature for all clinicians in British medicine. Moving audit from an occasional activity run by a few enthusiasts on national committees to a more general activity was controversial and the value of regular audit meetings is still debated. One can argue that:

- Compulsory audit meetings provide a cohesive element in an increasingly fragmented health service
- Communication between clinicians has improved as a result of audit
- Patients have benefited because the poor standard of care in some units has been highlighted and corrected
- Audit has resulted in mutual understanding of the roles of different professions and enhanced team building in clinical care
- Audit has enabled medicine to become more 'evidence based'

There is, however, a vocal group of clinicians who argue that these changes would have occurred anyway, that generating statistics is a waste of time, that audit is very expensive and that the resources would be better utilized elsewhere. The controversy is likely to continue.

Clinical audit needs to be used primarily as an educational activity. In North America, *necrotic audit* is a well-recognized phenomenon. This type of audit involves the repetitive public investigation, as a quality assurance exercise, of all critical incidents and deaths, many of which were unavoidable. The result is the generation of large volumes of paper and a bored disaffected audience.

Audit terms

A *clinician* is anyone involved with the provision of care to patients (or clients). Doctors, nurses, midwives, physiotherapists, radiographers and dieticians are all clinicians.

Uniprofessional audit involves a single professional group. For instance a group of specialists might agree appropriate guidelines for the introduction of a new drug or therapeutic technique. Because of their personal and medico-legal sensitivity, morbidity and mortality (M&M) meetings are usually uniprofessional.

Multidisciplinary audit involves several specialties within one profession working to solve a problem. Thus physicians, surgeons and anaesthetists may meet to discuss the peri-operative management of patients with a particular diagnosis.

Clinical audit involves clinicians from different disciplines debating topics and establishing guidelines. For instance, topics such as the management of wounds, care of pressure sores and treatment of acute pain can involve doctors, nurses, pharmacists and physiotherapists. Most successful audits will require managers to become involved if change is to take place.

Standards are mandatory directives.

Protocols indicate the best available practice, particularly in clinical care. Clinicians can ignore a protocol if they feel that there is good reason so to do, but must be able to justify their actions. Cardio-pulmonary resuscitation protocols are widely accepted and many aspects of nursing care are controlled by protocols.

Guidelines suggest, but do not demand, that a particular clinical course of action is followed. They are designed to assist clinicians dealing with relatively uncommon clinical or managerial problems.

Legal position

The courts in Britain have taken the view that the presence of a standard, protocol or set of guidelines does not absolve a doctor from using professional judgement when treating an individual patient. However, if something goes wrong it will usually be easier to defend a doctor who has treated a patient using commonly accepted principles than if a maverick treatment has been tried. When producing recommendations for treatment the term guidelines is preferred to protocol or standards.

Audit cycle (Box 8.4)

The audit cycle is a quality cycle.

1. Choose a topic.

2. The audit group should decide, on the basis of the available information, what is 'best practice'.
3. Clinical guidelines are constructed to reflect this practice.
4. If there is no information about what is happening locally at present, an audit study is undertaken to assess current practice.
5. At a subsequent meeting the audit group decides how far local practice is from the ideal and produces clinical guidelines to move the existing state closer to the ideal. Whenever possible a series of targets are designed to assist the process of change and indicators developed to show whether progress is being made towards the new ideal.
6. Some time after the guidelines have been introduced, the audit should be repeated to see whether there have been sustained improvements.

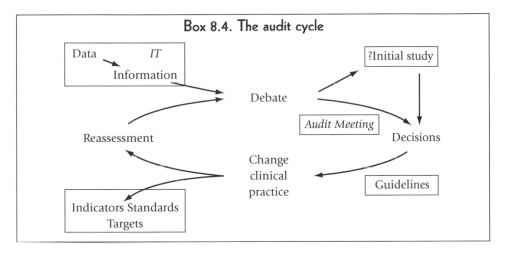

Box 8.4. The audit cycle

During the initial sequence of an audit cycle it is important to discuss ideal practice *before* finding out what is happening locally, otherwise the discussions may be coloured by attempts to maintain the existing state of affairs rather than looking for new solutions to old problems.

The audit process works well when used to assess routine clinical situations, such as the management of acute pain, or myocardial infarction. Guidelines can help clinicians deal properly with situations that are encountered less commonly — for instance managing acute anaphylaxis. *Integrated care pathways* in which the work of all the professions are co-ordinated can improve the efficiency of caring for patients undergoing routine major orthopaedic procedures. However the danger with the audit process is that a unit can become overwhelmed by too many poorly constructed guidelines. Senior staff then use these guidelines as an excuse to blame others for their own organizational deficiencies if something goes wrong.

Implicit in audit is the belief that one should always strive to do better. Complacent doctors do not see the point of audit, and rarely provide the best possible care for their patients. Health care is now so complex that all clinical and management staff need to be involved if care is to be altered and improved.

Collecting data

SKILL LEVEL 2

Early in your specialist training you may be asked to help collect data, either for a research project or for a clinical audit. When you first become involved you should concentrate on:

- Producing an effective data gathering tool
- Persuading people to co-operate and collect the data you need
- Turning the data into information
- Presenting the information you have obtained

Data gathering tools

Before starting, consider whether you ought to obtain permission for your study from the hospital ethics committee (p. 109); if unsure contact its chairperson. Next, find out if anyone in the hospital already collects the information you need. Clinical audit, information and quality assurance departments may be able to help you. They can offer advice on designing forms, using information systems, analysing data and presenting the results. They may also be able to provide you with a *download* of the information you want from the hospital information system. Check whether your hospital has any policies about the distribution of questionnaires; some trusts have developed a central system to ensure that staff and patients never get invited to take part in more than one study.

The simplest way to gather data is to design a *written questionnaire*. This is difficult. Questionnaires must be concise, and should preferably fit onto one side of A4. Write down the essential information that you need to know, and try to phrase unambiguous questions to obtain it. Then ask several people how they interpret what you have written. People will often find good reasons for misunderstanding your questions, so improve them. Apart from conventional written questionnaires, you can get people to fill in computer-friendly *forms* that can be scanned or optically mark-read, perform face-to-face *interviews*, or collect data directly onto a lap-top computer.

Hint: Forms can often be designed more easily by using a computer spreadsheet than a word-processing package.

Persuading people to co-operate

The best way to persuade people to co-operate with your study is to go and talk to them. A personal request is likely to be more effective than a circular. Try to persuade everybody of the value of your study. If you are planning to seek information from patients after discharge, seek their permission for you to contact them at home. Hospital questionnaires should never be sent unsolicited to a patient's home; they may cause embarrassment if relatives were unaware of the patient's visit to hospital. If you are doing a study which involves the completion of many questionnaires, it is essential that you keep track of the data and chase-up any missing or incomplete questionnaires regularly. People will complete your forms for a defined period of a week, or possibly even a month, but will get bored and give up if studies go on longer.

Analysing data

The simplest way to analyse data is to use a paper and pencil. This is quick and simple for small volumes of data, but impractical for larger studies. An effective way to analyse large amounts of data is to use a computer database or spreadsheet (see p. 56). A modern desktop computer will sort and count large amounts of data almost instantly, but each of the suitable programs is different and it is beyond the scope of this book to tell you how to use these tools.

Presenting the information

Once you know what you have found, you need to present the information appropriately. The graphical representation of information, the use of a computer presentation program and suggestions on how to present research findings are discussed in Chapters 7 and 9.

Completing a criterion-based clinical audit   SKILL LEVEL 3

You should assist with a criterion-based clinical audit during your training so that you:

- Understand the principles of criterion-based audit
- Are able to choose a suitable topic for audit
- Can gather information from various sources to determine best practice in that field
- Are involved in the formulation of audit criteria
- Can present information about your clinical unit in a diplomatic way
- Participate in the setting of guidelines and indicators resulting from the study

An audit project involves more than just collecting data, you need to be able to define the problems that your department faces, find acceptable solutions to them and negotiate the implementation of useful clinical guidelines. Box 8.5 summarizes the steps involved in completing a criterion-based audit.

Box 8.5. Summary steps involved in a criterion-based audit

Clinicians	Audit staff
Select topic for discussion	Conduct literature search
Define criteria for 'ideal' management	Identify sample from database Retrieve records Analyse and collate results

Discuss findings
Agree actions to move 'actual' state
  towards 'ideal' management
Produce and implement guidelines
Repeat study later to see if change has
  occurred	

Initial steps — selecting a topic

Find out who is in charge of audit in your department and agree upon a topic to be studied. Often, the most effective audits come from measuring simple things — for instance:

- Can working suction equipment be got to any acutely ill patient within 20 seconds?
- How many ward staff know the location of the nearest defibrillator?
- What proportion of prescriptions are legible and correct?
- Do trolleys tip?

Many departments prefer to look at more complex problems such as:

- How effectively particular clinical problems are dealt with
- How well different clinical teams communicate
- Whether costly drugs or blood products are being used appropriately

Establishing criteria

You now need to investigate the topic you have selected. Are there generally accepted views of best practice? Are there any existing scoring systems or questionnaires that help quantify the problem? Read the latest reviews on the topic and look up relevant papers. Find out if similar audits have been carried out in the past in your hospital (if this information is not on a computer database, ask your audit manager for copies of the hospital annual audit reports, which should list all past studies). Prepare for the initial audit meeting by producing simple overheads of the topic and the conclusions that you have reached as a result of your reading.

At the audit meeting you should aim to establish commonly agreed criteria for good practice. Try to get some impression of national statistics and what the local group would wish to see as standards. For instance you might agree that:

- 100% of all patients arriving in casualty should be triaged by an experienced nurse within 10 minutes of arrival
- 95% of all patients admitted with a fractured neck of femur should have their operation within 24 hours of admission
- No more than 3% of patients admitted for gynaecological day-case surgery should need to stay overnight

It can be very difficult to achieve a consensus. Some people will be keen to explain why changes cannot be made, rather than focusing on what targets should be sought and different ways of achieving these. A senior and experienced chairperson is a great help.

Preparing for the study

Once criteria have been agreed, you need to decide how to collect the data and how long the audit will take. Review what you learned at Skill Level 2 (pp. 98–99). Discuss your study with someone who understands the hospital information system. Usually the hospital information manager or audit co-ordinator will be able to help with obtaining notes, analysing them and turning the data into useful information. Discuss your needs before you embark on time-consuming donkey-work. It may be that most of the information you require is already available. Particularly in fields such as trauma and intensive care, existing scoring systems such as TRISS, or APACHE may be useful. Failing this you will have to develop a questionnaire and gather the data.

Presenting results

When you have gathered your data, you need to present it at another audit meeting. Start your presentation by reminding everyone of the criteria they accepted, then present your data. It may be that you simply confirm that all is well and you can all pat yourselves on the back and retire to coffee. Sadly, this is rarely the case and shortcomings will be exposed. Your aim now is to make the meeting produce some feasible and practical suggestions to improve things. To do this effectively you need to make sure that all relevant groups are represented. You may have to include managers, nurses or other clinical groups in your discussions. Very often the suggestions require new resources and are therefore difficult, if not impossible, to achieve. The ideal set of recommendations involves change in practice without change in resource. Furthermore it must be acceptable to nearly everyone concerned.

Aftermath

At the end of the meeting you should produce:

- A set of minutes recording criteria, findings and results
- Clear policies to improve the current condition
- Recommendations for a course of action
- An agreed implementation period after which the topic should be reanalysed to see if change has occurred.

Assessing the effectiveness of an audit meeting

Poor planning and presentation make some audit meetings a waste of time. They should be effective, educational, and entertaining. Audit itself needs to be audited and you can assess the value of your departmental audits using the criteria in Box 8.6.

Box 8.6. Auditing audit

- Was the meeting publicized in advance?
- Did most departmental staff attend?
- Were relevant topics discussed?
- Were common problems discussed?
- Did the discussion have an educational value?
- Were clear criteria established?
- Were all staff involved in the setting of these criteria?
- Did you learn anything?
- Will your practice alter as a result?

Evidence-based medicine

Evidence-based medicine is defined as: *the conscientious, explicit and judicious use of the best external evidence in making decisions about individual patients.* Audit requires a knowledge of 'best practice', but in many branches of medicine it is not clear what 'best practice' is. Vast amounts of research are performed, but results may conflict and the literature is biased by the tendency for editors to print papers that demonstrate positive findings, while rejecting those with negative results. Even slight publication bias can turn a random finding into a positive result if the studies are repeated. With so many journals now in print, it is difficult to obtain and evaluate all relevant papers pertaining to a topic.

To try to overcome this problem the *Cochrane collaboration* has been established. This is a group of specialists who select research topics, obtain all the papers published in a particular field, evaluate the merits of the trials, and combine the results using complex analytical tools such as meta-analysis to evaluate the evidence. Meta-analysis is the quantitative mathematical analysis of the results of separate research projects and is better than the more common qualitative review of a subject by an author, whose findings will almost certainly be affected by personal prejudices and the quality of the databases that are used to search for information.

Having determined which treatments are effective and which should be discarded, the findings can be distributed in the hope that they will form the basis of future medical practice. When satisfactory evidence about the merits of a particular therapy are lacking, then a research agenda emerges. Evidence-based medicine is not about rationing as it may well demonstrate that effective treatments are expensive while cheap treatments do no good, but the results should be presented in a form which allows doctors to determine the relative cost of their treatments per patient effectively treated.

In order to produce results in a form that means something to the average doctor, systematic reviews reported under the evidence-based medicine system are avoiding traditional ways of showing statistical likelihood, and instead are presenting information in new ways.

RRR, Relative risk reduction

RRR is a derivative of the type of statistics that most people are used to. In a trial, one group of patients might suffer a complication in 10% of control cases (C) and 3% of treatment cases (T). The RRR is $(C-T)/C$, in this case a 70% reduction. The problem with RRR is that it takes no account of the importance of the finding. For instance if a new treatment of a large group of patients reduced a complication from 100 to 30%, the finding would be very important, but a reduction from 0.001 to 0.0003% would have the same RRR value, but a much smaller clinical significance.

ARR, Absolute risk reduction

ARR simply uses the formula $(C-T)$ so that one can judge the effects of the treatment more easily. In the two examples above, $(C-T)$ for 100% to 30% is a 70% reduction, while for 0.001 to 0.0003% is a 0.0007% reduction. ARR values are usually small decimal numbers and are difficult to remember.

NNT, Number needed to treat

To make the figures easier to understand, the reciprocal of the ARR is quoted. 1/ARR is a useful figure because it is the number of patients that must be treated to produce one beneficial result. This is termed the number of patients needed to treat or NNT. By considering the benefits of the procedure, the NNT and the cost per treatment, it becomes possible to evaluate the cost-effectiveness of the procedure.

Other ways of using evidence to make judgements

There are other terms associated with measurement and quality which have greater relevance to managers than to clinicians.

Quality assurance

Quality assurance is a management process which ensures that there are properly defined systems for dealing with most common problems. Usually this involves establishing clearly defined and written policies so that all staff know what their responsibilities are, how problems should be dealt with and who is responsible for taking action. Activity within the organization can then be assessed against these criteria. This sounds like common sense and something that all organizations ought to have in place. The problem is that actually defining responsibilities can be enormously time-consuming, while establishing written policies for most eventualities produces huge amounts of paper. The process of discussing and establishing the quality assurance system is probably more important than the paperwork. A national standard, BS5750, can be applied for by organizations with effective quality assurance systems in place. External management auditors review the way that the organization works and its management systems. Many commercial companies aspire to this standard and some NHS units have fulfilled the requirements.

Departmental morbidity and mortality meetings should assess whether the individual care of patients has conformed to expected standards, protocols, guidelines and clinical expectations. As such, morbidity and mortality meetings are classified as quality assurance meetings rather than audit, because new policies rarely arise from the consideration of one patient.

Risk management

Risk management is increasingly important in medicine because litigation is becoming more common. It requires organizations to look at the work that they do and anything that places staff, patients or relatives at risk. Poor maintenance of the driveways, ineffective fire precautions, inadequate numbers of lifting aids and lack of induction policies for locum doctors would all be picked up by a risk assessor. Risk assessment is best performed by someone from outside the organization who has extensive knowledge of the problems and their possible solutions, but does not ignore them simply because they are mundane.

Monitoring systems

Effective organizations need to know how they are performing. Many hospitals have established quality assurance departments which receive information about what is going on throughout the organization. They deal with accident reports, patient complaints and compliments, and the results of surveys such as those by hygiene and fire inspectors. By gathering information about the way that systems work, patterns may build up. Well run wards gain plaudits and have only occasional problems, while less effectively managed parts of the organization tend to have a multitude of problems.

The value of quality initiatives

A lot of money has been spent on quality initiatives, and the medical audit program has required doctors to participate in regular audit meetings. Many clinicians feel that the money would have been better spent on patient care and that the time involved could have been better used dealing with clinical problems. Decisions taken at audit meetings are often ignored or take a long time to introduce. Despite a training that is supposed to emphasize the scientific aspects of knowledge, most doctors change their practice as a result of anecdotal or personal experience rather than evidence from large-scale trials. The way that audit was initially presented to the professions in the UK generated antagonism. In North America, the health care management organizations have produced their own 'care profiles' and have linked funding to what they perceive to be the most appropriate care. Such 'care profiles' can conflict with a clinician's personal beliefs about effective treatment. Large numbers of senior doctors therefore remain very sceptical about the value of quality initiatives.

It is important to balance this scepticism against the changes that have been seen in the British NHS since the 1989 White Paper. These changes include:

- More openness in the discussion of clinical problems
- Greater awareness of the need for team-based clinical care
- A more patient-centred rather than organization-based system of health care
- Increased use of day case facilities in a way that patients approve of
- Shorter waiting lists for many conditions

These changes reflect the demands of society as a whole, but have been brought about by fundamental shifts in the way that professionals see themselves and work together. Many changes in clinical practice, for instance the shift from in-patient to day case surgery, come about as a result of alterations in many fields of practice including:

- Better patient education
- New methods of patient assessment
- Better anaesthetic drugs
- New surgical techniques
- Improved post-operative pain relief
- Changes in the way patients are nursed
- Formation of improved links between community and hospital care

These changes have taken place because the work of many different professional groups has been co-ordinated. Audit and quality management systems are only part of this change, but they have been fundamental to its success.

A final thought
If clinicians do not audit and manage themselves, then someone else will do it for them, and this is likely to be a much less satisfactory solution.

9. RESEARCH

Objectives of this section

- to suggest how you can select a topic for research
- to describe the principles of obtaining ethical consent
- to indicate how to organize a research project
- to describe how to write and submit a research paper

Doctors do research for various reasons, the most common being:

- They want to understand more about research methods
- They need to improve their CV
- They have been recruited by a senior member of staff to assist with a study
- They want to find out more about a subject

Sadly, outside academic medicine, the last of these reasons is probably the least common. With the introduction of structured training in the UK, research has become a less important aspect of specialist training. However, candidates wanting to be short-listed for prestigious consultant posts will still need to have a strong research background.

Research skills

Some of the skills that can be learnt by participating in research are listed in Box 9.1. If you are trying to learn these skills by taking part in a project, your overall understanding of each skill will depend upon the amount of time and effort that your supervisors can find to teach you. An alternative, and possibly more effective way to learn about research, is to join a university course on research methodology, some of which result in a diploma or BSc degree.

Box 9.1. Research skills

- Selecting topics for research
- Literature searches
- Gaining ethical approval for a study
- Recruiting patients
- Acquiring practical research techniques
- Acquisition and interpretation of data
- Using information technology
- Being able to present research data
- Writing research papers

Selecting a topic for research

If your main aims are to learn research techniques and improve your CV by publishing some papers, you do not need to be fussy about the subject of your research. You should choose a subject in which:

- Your department already has a good research record
- Appropriate equipment, facilities and laboratory staff are available to support the research
- Suitable patients are fairly plentiful, and likely to stay in hospital for several days.

It also helps if:

- The study is a continuation of previous published work
- The main researcher/co-ordinator is still working in the department
- You have some interest in the subject!

A convenient way of learning research techniques, without requiring too much original thought, is to join an existing study. You may be able to participate in a long-term research project conducted by an academic department, or work with another researcher who has thought of a good idea for a study. Such collaborations can benefit both you, and other members of staff who have ideas but lack time to investigate them.

If you are really keen to initiate a completely new project, make sure you will be able to obtain willing senior advice and find a mentor who has experience of the research field. Research projects take time to set up and must be organized carefully. If you need additional equipment, or staff to help you during the study, you must apply well in advance for grants or loan of equipment. Logistic arrangements eat into the time you need for research. Only consider tackling a subject which will require you to develop new experimental techniques if you have plenty of time available — usually at least 2 years. Projects of this type are usually the subject of PhD theses and require specific funding.

Consider whether you want to do clinical research or a laboratory study. If your study involves patients, you must get ethics committee approval (see below). The easiest way to find out if your application is likely to succeed is to get informal advice in advance from a member of the ethics committee. Submit your application as early as possible, so that if objections are raised you will have time to make changes before you waste valuable research time. If you have a limited amount of time to do research, or if you can only perform your studies at a set time each week, try to make the scope of your study as broad as possible. It is always difficult and time-consuming to recruit patients. If you are too selective, your study will never be completed.

Laboratory or animal studies avoid the problems of patient recruitment, and it becomes much easier to organize your research time. However, animal research presents ethical dilemmas. Most experimental protocols will require that the animal is sacrificed at the end of the experiment. You will need an animal handling licence, and must be able to justify the loss of animal lives both to yourself and to others — some of whom may be passionately opposed to animal experiments.

As a consultant you can enjoy the luxury of undertaking research for its own sake, but as a trainee your object in doing research must be to get a publication in a peer-reviewed journal. Repeating previously published work or undertaking clinical research that has little or no clinical relevance is probably a waste of time. When you submit your paper the journals' reviewers will consider not only the study design, conduct and data interpretation, but also its relevance.

Once you have begun a project, you have an obligation to finish it. People have paid for your time and equipment, and patients have assisted you; they expect something worthwhile will come from the study. If you are running out of time, consider involving others. If you have bothered to start a project it is better to get it finished and published rather than drag it out so that it never gets finished or the researchers become bored. Although a larger number of names on a publication may appear to dilute the input of the individual, it will not stop it being published in a good journal. Delays may result in identical work being published by someone else first — very few research ideas are unique.

Getting ethical consent for human research

The Nazi atrocities perpetuated in the name of medical science (*BMJ* Dec 7 1996) demonstrated that ethical regulations were mandatory whenever human experimentation took place: 'Those involved in horrible crimes attempted to excuse themselves by arguing that there were no explicit rules governing medical research on human beings in Germany during that period...' Rules and monitoring are necessary to control doctors who, through obsession and fanaticism with or without scientific curiosity, want to perform experiments which go beyond the interest of the experimental subject.

Most scientific journals will publish articles only if the authors submit evidence that the study had formal approval by an ethics committee. This, and the fact that organizations which provide large sums of money for research, such as the Medical Research Council (MRC), demand ethics approval, help to police research (see also Chapter 13).

Applying for ethical consent
You must obtain ethical consent if your research involves humans or the use of human material (including foetal and embryonic tissue or material from the recently dead). In 1991 the Department of Health extended the remit of

ethics committees to cover any research undertaken on NHS premises, any subjects acquired via the NHS, or which involved information in present or past NHS notes. If you are unsure whether you need ethics committee approval for your research project, or your research is either on subjects or premises unrelated to the NHS, seek advice as failure to gain necessary ethical consent can lead to serious criticism later.

Usually, you need to apply to the Local Research Ethics Committee (LREC) for consent. LREC consent is valid only for their own hospital and you will need to apply separately if you want to conduct research at more than one site. To reduce the bureaucracy involved in gaining consent for multicentre trials, Multicentre Research Ethics Committees (MREC) are being established by the Department of Health and these will work with local committees to facilitate ethical reviews of studies which are to be undertaken in five or more localities. Ethical consent given by an MREC will be valid throughout the UK.

Ethics committee members are volunteers and the committee must have one medical person, one lay person (with no local trust connection), one male and one female. Other likely members include a pharmacist, a GP, a clinical nurse and a statistician. The actual number of people and their professional interests will vary from one committee to another. Meetings may take place monthly in a university hospital, but will be more infrequent in a smaller hospital. Processing an application can take anywhere from 1 to 6 months. Find out from the LREC secretary how often the LREC meets and the closing dates for applications.

Academic departments should have a copy of the application form either as a hard copy or on computer disk. If not, contact the LREC secretary. The LREC application form is lengthy and you will be expected to provide an understandable and legible summary of the work you plan, usually typewritten. The forms are designed so that the committee can satisfy themselves about four considerations:

1. *Beneficence* — are you doing research in the interests of your subjects or the population?
2. *Non-maleficence* — are you doing any harm?
3. *Rights* — the rights of all involved (subjects and researchers) must be preserved;
4. *Justice* — that resources are not unfairly spread as a result of research interests.

Completing the application form
Be prepared to spend several days preparing your application form. The actual form will take 2–3 hours to type, and considerable background information is required. Typical headings are listed in Box 9.2.

> ## Box 9.2. Headings used in ethical consent forms
>
> 1. *Details of applicants*
>   This consists of details of the applicant and other researchers — make sure your supervisor or head of department will be available to sign the form before the deadline for submission.
> 2. *Details of project*
>   The aims and objectives of the project must be outlined. It is worth spending time on this part of the form as it can be used as the basis for an abstract submission or form the outline of the introduction or discussion when you come to writing the project up.
> 3. *Recruitment of subjects*
>   Details of how they will be recruited and the information that they will be given.
> 4. *Consent*
> 5. *Drugs/medical devices*
>   You will be expected to have all the relevant details of experimental drugs or devices from the supplying company.
> 6. *Ionizing radiation*
>   If you plan to use ionizing radiation you will need to be a certificate holder.
> 7. *Details of interventions*
> 8. *Risks and ethical problems*
> 9. *Indemnity and confidentiality*

A checklist is usually supplied so that you can make sure you have submitted all the relevant documentation and do not run the risk of rejection due to a small oversight.

Failure to obtain ethical approval

Ethical approval is usually deferred rather than rejected out of hand. The most common reason for rejection is a badly written patient information sheet. Too often, doctors design information sheets that include complex medical terminology which is unlikely to be understood by a lay person. Take care to avoid this, but if this is the reason why approval has been withheld, it is easily corrected.

Trials that involve placebo drugs must be considered carefully; it is no longer acceptable to use a placebo as comparison for a new drug if a cheap and satisfactory alternative agent has already been shown to be effective and beneficial. A few applications are rejected because they are unethical, the risks outweigh the benefits to too great an extent.

Performing research

Obtaining funding, gathering equipment and obtaining outline ethical agreement are the initial stages of the project. Once you have agreement that the project is feasible you can move on.

Perform a power analysis

Power analysis is a statistical technique to enable you to determine how many individual studies you need to perform to prove your point. Highly effective treatments can be proved by studying small numbers of patients, but the efficacy of less substantial therapeutic changes can be validated only if you study a large group. The days of single researcher studies are nearly over; they are being replaced by multi-centre and international studies. Power analysis will not help if you do not know how effective your treatment is likely to be. Asking a statistician for help early in your study will probably save you much time and effort later.

Inform consultants and staff

It is important that all relevant medical and nursing staff are briefed about your study. Common courtesy requires you to tell them what your study is about, the reasons for it, any effects that it may have on the patients, and any procedural changes that may affect them. You must have the permission of the clinical consultants to study their patients. If you offer to give a small presentation on the subject of your research you can solve several problems at once. Make sure that clinical staff can contact you easily.

Documentation

Make sure you have prepared all the necessary information, consent and data collection forms. Back these up on computer disk. If you are not at ease with computers then now is the time to learn about word-processing, databases and a presentation package (see Chapters 5–7).

Research techniques

You may have to learn some clinical or laboratory skills. Practise these thoroughly before you start the main phase of your research project. Your results may be distorted if you are refining your methods during the initial studies.

Equipment

If your study involves the use of special equipment, ensure that it is working correctly and that you understand how to use it. You need to have access to a research technician who can help you maintain it.

Laboratory help

Contact any laboratory staff involved in the study. Ensure that they understand what you want. Make sure you know how specimens or samples should be collected and stored before examination or assay. This is particularly important if you will be working out-of-hours and having to store samples overnight or for a weekend.

Identify research times and staff availability

Try to identify times for performing studies that are convenient to all the team involved. However, it can be difficult to plan ahead now that fewer patients are admitted the night before an operation and many leave hospital soon after surgery.

Data collection phase of the study

Once the preliminaries are complete and you are ready to start collecting data, you should design a check list of things that you need for each study. For example:

- Patient consent
- Research team availability
- Additional staff information
- Equipment availability and function
- Specimen pots
- Data forms

Inevitably, as you gain experience, you will become slicker at performing the study, so it is sensible to have a few practice sessions before formally collecting data so that initial mistakes do not interfere with the experimental results. If you are working in a team, it is easier and more reliable to perform the same tasks each time. However, you do need to understand other people's jobs so that you can substitute for them if they are away.

At the end of each individual study:

- Make sure any specimens or samples are appropriately labelled, stored and sent to the lab for analysis
- Collect all the data forms and put them onto a database as soon as possible. Have a safe filing system for the originals
- Clear up and check your equipment ready for use the next time. Make sure that things are set up for the next study so that you can get going in a hurry if necessary
- Follow-up the patient and thank them

Other tips

Make the most of the times that you are not actively researching. Make some of the initial preparations for writing up. You can at least prepare some of the introduction and method. Keep up to date with the work that is being published in your field.

If you are doing full time research work, do not stick to one project. Have several on the go so that you always have something to work on. Even with the best will in the world, not all projects can be completed, and not all projects are publishable in peer-reviewed journals. Use your research effectively. Present your results as an abstract to a meeting or write it up for a local journal. All this experience is useful. Take advantage of your research time to do other things — write a review article or case reports, plan a presentation or give regular tutorials. Try to be proactive as it can be all too easy to let time slip away

Make sure that you record all references comprehensively — see the next section.

Writing a paper

Firstly decide which journal you would most like to publish your work. There is an unspoken pecking order for journals. You should aim for a peer-reviewed journal. This means that your work is reviewed by experts in that field who comment on your work and whether they feel it is worthy for publication as it stands, with modifications, or not at all. If your work is a continuation of previous research it makes sense to send it to the journal that published the earlier work.

If you are refused publication by a particular journal you can always submit to a less well-known journal, or non-peer-reviewed journal. This may have less kudos but at least you have not wasted all your efforts.

There is an unwritten code of practice with respect to publication which it is sensible to follow. If you have presented an abstract or poster of your work at a meeting then you should submit your work to the relevant body in the first instance. So, for example if you have presented at the Anaesthetic Research Society, you should submit to the *British Journal of Anaesthesia*. If the work is rejected outright you are then at liberty to submit it elsewhere. You must submit your work to only one journal at a time. This rule applies to presentations as well. You should not present the work in the same or similar form at more than one meeting, so choose the best and most appropriate venue.

Using the word-processor
With the invention of WYSIWYG programs even a novice can grasp the basics of word-processing. You should aim to get to grips with basic computer packages during your research time; this is certainly necessary before you start to do the writing up. No secretary will appreciate typing out draft after draft of illegible handwriting, and for speed and convenience you need to be able to do the writing yourself.

Writing up

Having decided where you would like to submit your work, read the relevant 'Guide to Contributors'. It will give you information about the basic rules of writing up, legal considerations and the preparation of the manuscript including presentation, formatting, figures, and illustrations.

It saves time and effort if you start writing in the correct format. If you are submitting work that follows on from a previously published study write in the same descriptive style. Obtain the earlier papers and read them. There is nothing to stop you imitating (this does not mean copying verbatim) the style for the *Summary, Introduction and Method* as they will inevitably be similar. If you have no previous experience of writing, use your ethics submission as the basis for the *Introduction and Method*. This will contain most of the relevant information. A lot of the initial writing of the paper can take place while you are collecting or analysing results. You will of course need to have completed analysis of the results before you write the discussion.

References

References are one of the biggest headaches of writing a paper. Gather together all the necessary references, read them and log them, ensuring that you record the whole reference in a standard format.

For each reference you should record:

- Authors' names and forenames — all of them
- Full title of article
- Journal name and official abbreviation
- Publication volume, issue number, date, start and finish pages.
- A brief summary of the paper

For books you should additionally record

- The names of the editors
- The edition
- The publishing company and their city
- The year of the publication

Careful recording of this information initially will save you having to return to your sources when you write your paper. A suitable computerized reference management program such as End Note™ enables you to insert references easily and to change their layout quickly if publishers have different formatting requirements. Inaccurate referencing is common and frustrates readers who want to look up to the original work. Be accurate.

Statistical analysis

Most research novices dread statistics, and few have enough knowledge to successfully attempt statistical analysis unaided. A research department should have a statistics expert available. Get help early. You ought to have got advice when setting up your study to ensure that your study groups were suitable (see p. 112). Go back to your expert to make sure that you select an appropriate method for analysing your results. Good statistical analysis makes it more likely that your paper will be accepted. A simple approach that gives you the result you want, but is not supported by valid statistics, is likely to be rejected by reviewers. Some journals now supply a statistical check-list so that they can be clear about the your analysis techniques. Failure to produce a statistically significant result does not invalidate your research, unexpected or negative results are sometimes worth publishing.

After the first draft

Once you have written a draft paper put it away for a few days and then go back to it. You will find that you approach it with new energy, and phrase construction and clarification become easier. Use 'spell check' to correct some of the mistakes you have not noticed. Now give it to a decent linguist to read and criticize. This is particularly important if English is not your first language. When you are happy with your version give it to the person over-seeing your research for final editorial comment before submitting it.

Before you submit the paper:

- Make sure you have complied with all the rules for contribution
- Check your referencing one last time
- Make sure you have a complete hard copy of your written work, results and illustrations
- Make sure the final draft is stored on both hard and backup floppy disks
- Send your work as requested (hard copy or disk) with a covering letter which includes details of your name and an address for correspondence. Remember you may not hear from the journal, apart from acknowledge-ment of receipt, for 3 months or so

Rejection

Reviewers like to receive legible, well-written papers with clear arguments. Typical reasons for initial rejection include:

- A study of no interest or relevance
- An inappropriate subject for the journal
- Poor English and grammar, making interpretation difficult
- Poor presentation and disregard of formatting
- Incorrect statistical analyses

If your work is returned, you should be given reasons for this in a letter from the editor. Read the comments carefully as they may be offering constructive advice and not represent outright rejection.

Proofs

If your work is accepted, you should be sent proofs of your work to check before publication. Do this carefully, including all the figures and references. Mistakes often occur during transcription from one type of word-processing package to another at the publishers. Proof-reading is tiring and boring. At this stage try not to read your text in sentences, instead read each word in isolation and look closely for spelling errors and duplicated words. Look at tables very carefully, paying attention to easily overlooked features such as decimal points and quantities. The printers will usually supply you with a set of the standard proof correction symbols. Ensure that you have completed the work in the required time or you will delay publication.

Copies

You may be entitled to a number of off-prints. These are useful as people may wish to study your work in future. You may receive requests for copies of your paper from overseas, but the habit of requesting papers seems to be declining as Internet and fax communications improve. Add your paper to your CV, making sure that the reference you quote is correct in every respect.

10. GETTING THINGS DONE

Objectives of this section

- to understand what management is about
- to understand how to set priorities in your organization
- to take part effectively in committees
- To understand the basics of budgets

Management

Management is about organization and vision. A manager takes a long-term view, seeking to improve the overall efficiency of the organization, taking into account changes in customer/patient demands, financing, politics and technology. Good managers do not demand constant upheaval, but try to ensure that their organization remains innovative. Effective management reduces confrontation by good communication, although there will be occasions when change requires confrontation because of the inertia of established systems.

Administration, in contrast, consists of keeping things ticking over smoothly. Good administrators are extremely valuable and much under-rated. A person who organizes a duty rota without causing crises or bad feeling, or a clerk who ensures that patient notes are always available for out-patient clinics makes everybody's life easier and improves efficiency.

The health service reforms of the early 1990s increased the importance of management in the NHS. Many training courses in management techniques are available; doctors can, and probably should, attend one. However, management is mostly about dealing with people. Courses and degrees may improve your understanding of what managers can and should do, but will not necessarily improve your ability to influence other people. This section explains some of the mechanisms used to manage a hospital.

Running the NHS

In many ways, managing an NHS Trust is more complicated than managing a commercial company. Business targets are usually straightforward; increased profits result from producing larger numbers of better quality products at a lower price. Industries can invest when they are making a profit and can transfer surplus funds into reserves to protect against recession. In contrast, National Health Trusts operate within stringent financial controls, profit is not permitted and spare money cannot be saved.

Healthcare managers have to take other factors into account. Most individuals are not particularly interested in the quality of health services until they or a family member falls sick; they may then become passionately involved. The press loves stories about health, provided they are about 'breakthroughs', misdiagnosis, or mistreatment. Television images of hospitals bear little resemblance to reality, but govern peoples' perceptions. Priorities in health care are determined more by politics, emotion and pressure groups than by dispassionate analysis. A very rare problem that gets media attention, for example the abduction of a baby from a children's ward, can mean that large amounts of money are spent to prevent it happening again, while serious day-to-day deficiencies in services are neglected.

Paying for things

Many British doctors feel uncomfortable when dealing with money matters and think that money and patient care should be kept far apart. But staff and supplies must be paid for, and the NHS is given a finite sum of money each year by the government. Government in turn has to balance its books and can only spend what it receives from taxes and other revenues. For the past two decades, people have voted for parties of low taxation, and public services have felt the pinch. Given these constraints, it is inevitable that health care will be rationed by one means or another, and doctors have to play their part in rationing by helping to set priorities.

Planning

The planning cycle

To employ its budget effectively, an organization must plan. Such plans may be:

- *Strategic plans* with long-term aims or ambitions that take account of foreseeable changes in technology, demographics and demand over the next decade. A strategic plan enables an organization to decide what aspects of care it wants to concentrate upon, and to produce a 'wish-list' for the future. However, such plans are time-consuming to produce and rarely come to fruition in the anticipated way.

- *Business plans* which look forward 1 or 2 years. They show how money will be spent and so all proposals must be planned and priced. The annual round of business planning is an exercise in priority setting. Everyone is invited to suggest how their service might be improved (this often involves several expensive proposals) and where savings might be achieved (a less popular aspect). When finance is tight, a lot of time can be wasted putting forward proposals that are eventually rejected, however desirable they may be. Attempts are made to match anticipated income with expenditure and, eventually, a balanced budget for the next year is produced. The trust business plan is then negotiated, so that the aims of the purchasers match those of the providers. In reality the plan is usually disrupted by crises such as: an excessive number of winter medical admissions, changed political priorities, or the unexpected breakdown of an expensive piece of equipment.

- *Budgets* govern what each service can achieve. The overall income of the trust is divided and handed down to the service managers. Each service must work within very tight financial constraints. The budget balance at the end of each year is supposed to be within 0.5% of target and spare money can rarely be transferred from one year's accounts to the next. Profit is not allowed. The workload of the organization is constrained by these cash limits and managers may lose their jobs if there are serious budgetary problems.

Much time is consumed by this financial planning, but the health service is not a private company in that no major health provider in the NHS can be allowed to cease operating through bankruptcy. Thus a serious overspend usually results in a change in management and a cosmetic re-organization, not the immediate closure of a big hospital.

Establishing priorities

The production of a *mission statement* can be a valuable exercise in deciding strategic priorities within an organization or department. The entire department can consider such questions as:

- Is the department concerned primarily with offering a good clinical service, or are teaching and research thought to be important, despite the reduced clinical efficiency and increased costs that these engender?
- Which sub-specialties does the department wish to promote?
- Is everyone in the department to be involved in all aspects of the organization, or will a few people with a particular interest take on specific roles in for instance audit, teaching and management; if so, how will this extra work be recognized?
- Does the department wish staff to have a role in national and regional decision making processes despite the fact that this will take senior staff away from the department and reduce the amount of time they can teach and look after patients?
- Are good working conditions and a reasonable home-life for the staff important or secondary to clinical priorities?

Issues such as these have been ignored in the past, but are becoming increasingly important as budgetary control over doctors' work becomes tighter. Discussing these issues can be worthwhile, even if no firm conclusions are reached. Trying to embody the principles in a one or two sentence mission statement is a rather less valuable exercise, while exhibiting the result in a picture frame will impress fewer people still, particularly if the stated objectives are never fulfilled.

Business plans

The annual business planning cycle is supposed to make each department reassess its resources and aims regularly. There are two views of business plans: they are an effective way to plan for the future, or they are time-wasting procedures not worth the paper they generate. Doctor's views are governed by whether their ideas can be put into practice and this, in turn, is governed by the financial health of their trust.

A business plan is concerned with what, how, and when. The components of a typical business plan are shown in Box 10.1. Once the current position has been reviewed, the business plan should look to the future and consider:

- Possible developments — their merits and costs
- Possible savings that can be made to permit developments
- Long-term aims and objectives

Box 10.1. Components of a typical business plan

- The structure of the department
  who organizes what and how?
  how are things paid for?
  who is responsible if something goes wrong?
  are there appropriate clinical and managerial policies?
- Staffing
  are the facilities in the department adequate?
  are numbers correct?
  is the balance between specialists and trainees correct?
  are there enough support staff?
- Customer profile
  who are the stakeholders in the system?
- Service profile
  who is the department trying to serve?
  is it doing so effectively?
- Financial analysis
  is the income adequate?
  where does the money come from?
  can investment be attracted, revenue increased, or savings made?
- Quality and audit
  are effective quality assurance mechanisms established?
- Service
  is the department providing a good quality service to its customers and
    stakeholders?
- SWOT analysis
- Plans
- Developments and costs

The business plan should conclude with an action plan to bring about these changes.

Marketing

Marketing is sometimes equated, incorrectly, with advertising. Marketing is:

- Identifying need
- Discovering what customers, consumers or patients want
- Analysing how the current service is provided
- Seeing how the users of the service would like it altered or improved
- Producing plans to match demand with supply

Before a development is included in a business plan, a department must find out whether its proposal will help other parts of the organization and whether patients want it. Marketing involves identifying *stakeholders*, that is anyone who is affected by the service (Box 10.2). Senior management of a health organization must be aware of the demands of all these groups when planning changes. Attempts to change the provision of a service will usually fail if patient groups, community health councils and local politicians oppose it. At departmental level, it is important to be aware of the pressures that stakeholders exert on the running of a service: for instance, a plan to change a consultant's operating session from one day to another will have knock-on effects throughout the organization.

Box 10.2. Stakeholders

- Patients/clients/customers — either as individuals or through the Community Health Council
- Relatives of these individuals
- General practitioners
- Other clinicians of all professions and support staff
- Other hospitals
- Outside suppliers
- District purchasers
- The National Health Service Executive
- Local and National Politicians
- Pressure groups and charities — particularly those funding or representing specialist services

---

SWOT analysis

The SWOT analysis is useful at both a personal and organizational level for analysing the present situation and foreseeable changes. The initials stand for four headings: strengths, weaknesses, opportunities and threats.

Strengths are the forces working in your favour; *weaknesses* are the factors working against continuing progress or maintenance of the present state.

Opportunities are possibilities for change and improvement, while *threats* may prevent these changes occurring. A SWOT analysis can make it easier for you to determine which of your goals you are likely to achieve and so enable you to prioritize the developments in your business plan.

Attaining your goals

The ability to manage effectively and so achieve your objectives, depends upon:

- Knowing what you are doing already, and potentially could do (*information*)
- Understanding what other people want and gaining their support (*marketing*)
- Deciding which options to select (*SWOT analysis*)
- Selecting what you can achieve most easily (*prioritization*)
- Becoming involved in the decision-making process and influencing it (*participation*)
- Making sure that you can obtain the necessary funds to achieve your goals (*influence*)
- Obtaining funding, and then using your budget in the most effective way (*budgeting*)

Committees

Some committees are established with a single specific task in mind, for example to plan a conference, and then disband when the task is complete. Others are regular advisory bodies, for instance recommending what equipment should be purchased. Larger committees often exist only to inform and disseminate information, and become mere talking-shops. Finally, the purpose of some committees gets lost in the mists of time and, though their members may not realize it, their discussions are pointless as no one pays them any attention. Your ability to achieve your management goals is likely to depend upon how effectively you perform at meetings and thus you need to learn how committees function.

Structure of a committee

When a committee is formed the members must know why they are there, what job they have to do and to whom they have to report. Committees rarely have executive powers, though the chair or other individual members do sometimes have the power to implement decisions. More commonly, the views of the committee are summarized and transmitted back to a parent body where they may be accepted or rejected.

The official role of the committee is stated in its *terms of reference*. A committee has a *chair*, usually a deputy who acts if the chair is absent and a *secretary*. The secretary records the decisions of the committee in the *minutes*;

necessary so that time is not wasted repeatedly covering the same ground. The terms of reference may also define other members of the committee and the *quorum*, or minimum number of members who must be present for the committee to be officially constituted.

Joining a committee

Most people will feel flattered when invited to join a committee. But think:

- What is the committee seeking to achieve?
- How is it going to achieve these goals?
- How often does it meet?
- How is work distributed amongst the members of the committee?
- Who are the other members and what groups do they represent?
- Why have I been asked and how can I contribute?

The chair should be able to answer these questions succinctly, and additional information should be available by studying the terms of reference of the committee and, if it has met before, recent minutes. Beware of joining committees with little reason for existing, or when you are expected a fill a token role because someone in the distant past thought it a good idea to have representation from your interest group.

Once you have joined the committee find out how it works. Committees can be boring and mundane, but may be fascinating manifestations of complex power broking. Often members statements are coded and the nuances of the speaker must be understood. Everyone ought to be striving for a common goal, but this cannot be guaranteed. You must decide whether to participate actively and influence decision-making, or simply observe and contribute occasionally.

Attending a meeting

The chair should send out an agenda and relevant papers well in advance. The agenda gives structure to the discussion and usually follows a standard order:

- *Introductions and apologies*. If you are absent, your inclusion in the list of apologies allows you to dissociate yourself from an unpopular decision if ructions develop subsequently.
- *Signing minutes of the previous meeting*. If you believe that your opinions have been wrongly represented in the minutes, write to the chairman before the meeting and ensure that your objection is noted.
- *Chair's remarks*. The chair informs the committee about what has happened since its last meeting and sets the scene for current discussions by providing background information.
- *Matters arising from previous business*. Progress concerning previously discussed topics is discussed within the committee
- *Main business*. New topics for discussion are included in this phase of the meeting. Properly produced briefing papers enable all committee mem-

bers to contribute to the discussion. A clear plan of action ought to emerge, even if this is simply to postpone further discussion while more information is sought. Invited guests contribute during this phase of discussions.

- *Reports from sub-committees.* Large committees tend to sprout offspring. The reports of the sub-committees may be valuable, but major topics raised by them should be discussed under main business as the enthusiasm of most members is waning by this stage.
- *Any other business.* This stage must be strictly controlled by the chair. A well-recognized ploy is to raise a crucial matter late in the day when a lot of the committee has left. A wise chair will reject this ploy and invite the member to table the topic as main business at the next meeting. AOB is sometimes used to make political statements representing the views of a particular interest group.
- *Plans for future meetings.* Some committees have a fixed programme of meetings, for instance, the first Friday of a month. This is sensible for big and busy standing committees, but may be less appropriate for smaller working parties whose patterns of meetings should be flexible to ensure each meeting is as efficient as possible and that everyone can attend. Either way, the date and time of the next meeting must be clearly defined so that committee members can schedule it.

Chairing a committee

Committees succeed only if they have an effective chair. The chair decides the agenda and ensures that it is relevant and manageable. Committee members must be aware which issues are contentious and given adequate time to discuss them. This requires preparation, so that the chair is aware of the general sentiments of his committee and is able to encourage debate.

The chair must control meetings. All statements are made 'through the chair'; that is, members of the committee should talk only when invited to by the chair, a rule that prevents anarchy and several simultaneous conversations. If possible (and it is often very difficult), the chair should ensure that discussions remain relevant and succinct. Irrelevancies should be rejected. Important side-issues should be considered as a separate item on the agenda either at the next committee meeting, or under 'any other business'. At the end of each item on the agenda, the chair ensures that everyone has been given the opportunity to speak, and then summarizes the committee's decision so that it can be clearly minuted by the secretary.

After the committee is over the chair and the secretary must produce minutes which are a fair representation of the discussions. They must then ensure that the decisions are acted upon. Some committees produce an annual report that enables members of the committee to see what has resulted from their efforts. If little has been achieved, the committee should consider whether it should still exist; but tangible results are not the only reason for a committee to exist. Its role in allowing communication and understanding between groups with disparate views may be just as important.

Budgets

If you successfully persuade other people to fund your plans, you will have to manage the money that you receive. Budgets are *capital* or *revenue*.

Capital budgets

Capital budgets buy material goods: buildings, instruments or expensive bits of equipment such as X-ray machines. In turn, these budgets are designated for major or minor purchases.

Major capital funds are required for projects costing over one million pounds. Government approval is needed before a trust embarks on a project of this magnitude and the money may come from central NHS funds or be raised from private sources such as banks or industry through the Private Finance Initiative (PFI). Regardless of the source of funding, a proportion of the amount spent must be repaid each year in *capital charges*, which are similar to mortgage repayments. Capital charges are repaid from revenue funds and their cost must be included in your annual revenue budget.

Minor capital funds are used to purchase equipment costing from a few thousands, to tens of thousands of pounds. Individual trusts have discretion to purchase equipment in this price range and fund certain projects each year on the basis of need. Much of these budgets will be needed simply to replace obsolete or worn out equipment, and new medical devices may not be given a high priority.

Charities are often willing to pay for high-profile new equipment, but this equipment may require servicing, expensive disposable items, or staff to be trained and paid. These expenses need to be covered and some trusts require the charity to fund the revenue costs for a time before they will accept the equipment. Beware of the manufacturer who offers you a piece of 'free' equipment, such as an infusion pump; you will usually discover that the pump requires dedicated infusion sets only obtainable, at a premium, from a single supplier. If buying equipment from charitable funds it is usually better to pay the capital cost but ensure that the equipment can be maintained using cheap, readily available, disposable items.

Revenue funds

Revenue funds cover routine charges: salaries, maintenance costs, estate costs and disposable equipment costing under about £1000. They are the running costs of an organization. If you hold a budget, you are required to manage it so that it is not overspent at the end of the financial year but, as you will not be able to carry funds forward from one financial year to the next, there is little point in underspending. Indeed, a large underspend will result in a reduction in your budget next year on the grounds that you clearly received more than you needed. You may be able to transfer money between revenue and minor capital budgets and surplus revenue therefore usually gets spent at the end of the year in a spate of buying desirable, but not essential, equipment.

When running a revenue budget, a budget holder must liaise regularly with their business manager and accountant. Errors in revenue budgets are common and multiply with time. The account sheet will usually list: the actual amount spent in the past month, the overall spend in the present financial year, the planned spend for these periods and the difference between the two measures. Catches in revenue budgets include:

Salary costs

Usually budgeted at the mid-point of the salary scale for that group of staff and include a factor equal to approximately 15% of the persons salary to cover *on-costs* such as National Insurance and pensions. The use of mid-point salary means that if you always receive registrars early in a training rotation, you will have a consistent budget surplus as they will be paid at a lower rate than anticipated, while a department which only trains experienced registrars will note a consistent deficit. Paying locums to cover sickness or maternity leave will also cause an overspend, unless these factors are anticipated in your budget. In big departments the effects average out, but smaller budgets can run into problems if staff turnover is low and people move up their salary scales, or there is a bout of sickness.

Top slicing

Some money may be automatically removed from your budget to pay common costs. In some trusts, removal expenses and study leave are paid by top-slicing departmental budgets.

Re-charging

On some schemes, doctors are paid by a single trust throughout their training; that trust re-charges other trusts for the salary, removal and study leave expenses incurred when they work elsewhere. Thus some money may be automatically transferred each month from your budget. At some point, the principles for calculating the charges incurred by top slicing and recharging will have been negotiated by your trust finance department. However, the reasons for some of the deductions may been forgotten: accountants change as do management and educational structures. It is worth checking if the correct amounts are being removed from your accounts.

Estate costs

About a third of the cost of running a hospital is taken up with estate costs. These include building and ground maintenance, heating, lighting, rates, catering, engineering and portering. Trusts have different methods of distributing these costs between out-patients, day-cases and in-patients. Variations in the way these expenses are distributed largely account for the different amounts hospitals charge for the same procedure.

Accrual

To prevent overspending, the cost of an item is deducted from your budget when you order it. The money involved is thus hidden from you, even though it may be some time before the trust is obliged to pay its supplier. This early adjustment of budgets is termed accrual. Keep your budget up-to-date and ensure that money is refunded if goods are not delivered.

In summary: budgets are complicated, doctors need help to run them and need to keep their wits about them.

11. BEGINNING A CONSULTANT JOB

Objectives of this section
- to explain the consultant contract
- to describe some problems that may be encountered on appointment to a consultant post
- to discuss the role of consultant as team leader
- to explain how to write a reference
- to outline how to set up a private practice

Doctors spend about a third of their professional career as trainees. Once appointed a consultant, most will remain in one hospital for the rest of their career, so it is important to find a job that is enjoyable and challenging. The factors that must be considered when selecting consultant jobs were discussed in Chapter 1.

The consultant contract

Consultant contracts are held by NHS Trusts and each trust is able to set its own terms and conditions of service. A consultant contract contains three components:

- *Fixed sessions* — which the consultant must attend, as they involve resource allocation by the trust. Clinic sessions, operating lists and ward rounds are typical fixed session duties
- *Flexible sessions* — work that can be done at any time and requires few resources. The doctor is paid for this work, but does not have to state when the work will be done. Non-clinical duties including management, teaching, audit, administration, and committee work are fitted into the flexible sessions
- *On-call* commitment — reflected in the allocation of a certain number of flexible sessions

Consultants have to produce a *job plan* detailing their fixed sessions and sometimes including details of their use of other time. Most trusts still use the national terminology of full-time, maximum part-time and part-time employment. A *full-time contract* requires 11 notional half days (NHDs), or 37.5 hours a week committed to the NHS. Each NHD is 3.5 hours and an NHD is not equivalent to a theatre or clinic session, which is usually longer. Full-time consultants on typical contracts may earn from private practice sums no more than 10% of their total NHS earnings. Most newly appointed consultants begin on a full-time contract.

If you earn more than 10% of your salary in private practice you must, after 2 years, become a *maximum part-time consultant*. In return for dropping one NHD and an eleventh of your salary, you can undertake unlimited private practice provided that you fulfil all your NHS commitments. Maximum part-time consultants usually work the same number of fixed NHS sessions as their full-time colleagues. *Part-time contracts* are usually accepted by clinicians with domestic commitments, or those approaching retirement. They include fewer than 10 clinical sessions, private practice can be undertaken.

Contracts may be open-ended or fixed term. The contract will specify terms of service such as annual, professional and study leave and, although most contracts remain based upon the 'Whitley Council' terms negotiated before trusts took over management of their consultant staff, it is becoming more common for newly appointed consultants to negotiate their contracts of employment. Most trusts do not want to create friction by having each member of the senior staff on a widely different contract, so removal expenses and the increment on the pay scale at which you begin your contract are the features that are most likely to be negotiable. Colleagues and professional associations can give advice on what is fair and reasonable. It is sensible to seek the advice of an industrial relations officer of the BMA before accepting a contract.

The open-ended 'professional' contract has been satisfactory for the past 40 years, but fits less well with modern industrial practice. New contracts may be introduced which define responsibilities more closely and specify the amount of time that a doctor spends on:

- Clinical work
- On-call and emergency work
- Continuing medical education (CME)
- Education and teaching
- Management and administration
- Research

Such contracts might reflect more closely the different workloads of different specialties.

Consultant salaries

Consultants receive a basic NHS salary based upon the number of NHDs in their contract. They may, if they wish, earn fees from private practice and the contractual arrangements for this have just been discussed.

Earnings from other sources such as writing legal reports, or performing medical examinations for life insurance are termed category 2 work. This income does not result in reclassification of a consultant from full-time to maximum part-time under the 10% rule. Category 3 earnings come from waiting list initiatives and other extra-contractual work performed for GP fundholders. Schedule 3 earnings do count towards the 10% limit unless special arrangements have been negotiated.

The health service recognizes that some doctors contribute more than others and once you have reached the top of the consultant pay scale you will be eligible for additional trust *discretionary* pay awards or national *merit* awards. Each year eligible consultants are invited to submit a summary of their local, regional, national and international contributions. Each trust is required to make a minimum amount of money available equivalent to 0.25 discretionary points per eligible consultant per year. Doctors can be awarded up to five discretionary points. Regional and national committees allocate the B, A and A plus awards. Discretionary point committees include both doctors and managers, the higher awards are decided by medical committees. Inevitably, these awards are controversial, and the system can de-motivate doctors whose work remains unrecognized.

Getting started

Although your clinical workload may appear light, and you may have more spare time than during your registrar job, your first weeks as a consultant will probably be stressful. Everyone is judging your performance. New relationships need to be forged with trainees, nurses, managers and support staff. Clinical responsibilities increase steadily and can no longer be left behind at the end of the working day, because consultants are responsible for continuing patient care. Large volumes of mail arrive, some of which matters but most of which does not, and you may not be able to tell which is which. Medical students and post-graduate trainees need to be taught. You may feel isolated and you will not have the network of contacts that will eventually enable you to work efficiently. Your stress levels will decrease only when your confidence grows and you feel comfortable in your work.

New consultants can feel that, at the top of the ladder, they have no one to turn to for help. This is never true. Value the clinical skills and experience of your colleagues and trainees. Do not be afraid to ask for assistance, most people are flattered to be asked for their opinion and will not think any the less of you for asking. Beyond clinical medicine, most hospitals have 'elder statesmen' whose political judgements are widely respected, they should be consulted if you need your colleagues support to persuade management to accede to a request.

Induction
Hopefully, you new employer will provide you with an information pack as described in Chapter 1. If not, you will have to sort things out yourself.

Office facilities

The least you should expect is share of an office, a desk, a filing cabinet, a telephone and an appropriate amount of secretarial time. Computers, faxes, research laboratory space and your own secretary may be harder to come by, and you should be able to see that they exist before you believe the bland promises of a manager who may have moved on between the time of your appointment and the time you take up your post.

Technical requirements

Be quite clear early on what you need to do your job and ensure that it is all available. There are usually funds to enable a newly appointed consultant to buy some necessary equipment, but if it is not purchased right away you may have to wait a long time, competing with the conflicting priorities of all your colleagues.

Getting to know people

Attending committees and visiting the post-graduate centre will help you build up your network of contacts. In the early stages, be circumspect about taking on too many responsibilities, but participating in some hospital politics will enable you to discover how to influence people.

Moving house

An additional consideration for a new consultant is where to live. Factors to consider are:

- *Cost* — difficult as consultants who establish private practice may have a considerably greater income 5 years after appointment. A huge mortgage is a gamble and adds to personal stress
- *Education* — the distance to private schools, or the need to live within the catchment area of a good state school should be considered
- *Distance to hospitals* — living close to your places of work will save weeks of travel over the years. Many trusts specify that you should live within 10 miles, or 30 minutes travel time of the hospital; but may be lenient if you have reasons for living further away
- *Practising from home* — some consultants see their private patients at home. Their house must be suitably designed and accessible by public transport
- *Comfort* — your family must enjoy living in their home

Many newly appointed consultants prefer to rent, or move initially to a smallish house and relocate after a few years when they know better what they want and can afford.

Arriving

After a few weeks people start asking you for help and although the paper-work in the in-tray increases consistently, at least you know which bits to ignore and which to send on to someone else. You have arrived; now all you have to do is put up with it for the next 30 years! Some doctors get quite depressed at this stage. For 10 or 15 years they have devoted themselves to becoming a consultant; achieving it can be an anti-climax. With the attainment comes the realization that life hasn't really altered too much: medicine is still hard work and the pressures are different, not diminished. Future challenges will be set by your own ambitions.

The clinician as leader

Consultants are no longer, if they ever were, authoritarians who achieve what they want by shouting. They are part of teams providing care for patients, though their skills and experience will mean that members of the team look to them for leadership.

As the clinical team leader, the priorities of a consultant rub off on his staff. A courteous, well-organized, prompt, demanding autocrat is likely to attract staff who also approve of these characteristics. A less-structured personality is likely to attract a different group of staff. It is a useful exercise to decide what standards you regard as important and then ensure that your staff know you think they matter.

Until the early-1980s the main structure in British hospital medicine was the clinical 'firm'. A firm was led by a hospital consultant who was responsible for the total care of (usually) his patients. He was free to organize his workload, manage resources and teach his trainees more or less unconstrained by external influences. Usually his patients were nursed on a small number of wards and the sisters on these wards knew how he wanted his patients treated. It was a simple and effective administrative system, though one entirely dependent upon the personality and clinical acumen of the clinician and senior staff.

The health service is now more complex. The factors that ended the firm system were:

- Cost pressures, which led to a reduction in bed numbers and patients from one firm becoming scattered throughout hospitals
- Reductions in the length of patients' stay in hospital, and in particular the development of specialist short-stay units serving large numbers of consultants
- Reductions in trainees' hours-of-work so that each firm no longer provides continuous care for its patients
- Increasing specialization, with the introduction of complex technical procedures, means that one consultant can no longer offer comprehensive care even in their designated specialty

- The development of specialized nursing posts, for instance as colostomy nurses or in palliative care teams, to match the demand of patients for improved information, care and counselling
- The increasing importance of the work of other professions, including physiotherapists, occupational therapists, and social workers in ensuring successful and timely discharge of patients
- The requirement by management to match patient care to the available contracts and resources. Managerial demands to control the waiting list and complete the designated contract may conflict with the clinical priorities perceived by the medical and nursing staff.

As a result, hospital medical care, as well as care in general practice, has increasingly required people to work in teams, where the actions of many separate individuals must be co-ordinated effectively. While consultants are responsible for the actions of their medical staff, they have no direct authority over the nurses or paramedical staff who assist in patient care. Each professional group in the NHS has its own governing body and individuals are responsible both to their controlling professional bodies and to their local management. A doctor cannot order a nurse or paramedic to do a task that conflicts with their code of practice or local management policies. Thus the interactions of hospital teams are far more complex than in business where everyone is ultimately responsible to a single chief executive. This anarchic organization has worked adequately over the years as most staff in the health service have tended to see their common aim to be helping patients. Some managers imported from commerce have failed to understand the complexity of the situation and have disrupted organizations by attempting to impose a rigid line-management system on all professional groups.

Authority and delegation in clinical teams
Qualified doctors are responsible for their actions, while consultants are responsible both for the actions of their clinical team and for the continuing care of patients. If a trainee undertakes a procedure of any type without informing a senior, they become wholly responsible for their actions, but if a more senior doctor is informed, then that senior becomes responsible for subsequent actions and may have to justify the action if the decision to delegate the task to the trainee proves unwise.

The situation can be more complicated than this: if the consultant believes that the trainee has been properly taught and the trainee is happy to proceed, then most of the responsibility for future actions returns to the junior. The final twist occurs if the consultant delegates responsibility without really knowing how skilful the trainee is; this can be regarded as inappropriate delegation if something subsequently goes wrong. When more than one clinical specialty is involved in the care of the patient the situation can become even more complicated. The courts have suggested that surgeons are at fault if they do not respond to inaction on the part of an anaesthetist during a crisis, while anaesthetists have a responsibility to act if incompetent surgery is being performed.

Delegation occurs every day at all levels of medicine. A house officer may ask a medical student to do an electrocardiogram. Delegating this task may be done as part of the student's education, which is wholly commendable, or as a way of lightening a heavy personal workload, which may be inappropriate if the student already knows how to produce an ECG and should be learning other skills. Successful delegation of the educational task requires that the student knows where to find the ECG machine, how to work it, how to discuss the procedure with the patient, and know how to interpret the result, albeit at a basic level. Delegation and the assumption of authority that it brings are often educational, but as the complexity of the delegated procedure becomes more complex, the process becomes more difficult. It is often much slower and more nerve-wracking for seniors to try to train novices in a technical branch of medicine than to complete the tasks themselves. The ability to delegate is an essential part of teaching, but is a skill that some people never learn.

Writing a reference

Consultants are regularly asked to give references, and soon after your appointment a trainee will make this request to you. You should take great care when writing references, an incautious phrase can blight a career.

Principles

References are a long-established part of the appointments process, but the value of their content varies. Usually doctors are keen to help their trainees by writing references, and it is very satisfying to be able to advance the career of a competent doctor. Occasionally you may think that a trainee is incompetent. Your choice is then either to refuse to write a reference, or to a write a damning one. The latter requires very careful thought and should be chosen only if you have firm evidence on which to base your assertions.

In medicine there has been a tradition of using references to damn with faint praise. When you begin to write references it is probably wise to agree to provide them only for those doctors who you feel able to support wholeheartedly, and to suggest that staff whose abilities you doubt look elsewhere. If you lack confidence in your counselling skills, you are not obliged to explain your reasons. Later, as a departmental director or an educational supervisor, you may not have this option, but you then have a duty to sit down with the candidate and discuss what you are going to write and why.

A reference should be succinct and yet cover all the aspects of a trainee's performance that the appointments panel wants to know about. It should try to paint a picture of the candidate's worth, skills and personality. When you first write a reference, show your draft to a senior colleague who has a lot of experience of interview committees, and get advice on how your comments will appear to the panel.

Some interview panels are issuing structured reference forms, asking the referee to grade skills. This type of reference assumes a dispassionate honesty that is not widespread in medicine! An honest assessor in a big hospital with top class trainees may grade a wholly competent candidate worse than the marks given to an average trainee from an unpopular peripheral hospital where few good trainees apply. Doctors often grade equivalent candidates differently. Unless you have considerable experience of assessment and appraisal mechanisms structured references should be treated with suspicion; too dispassionate an honesty may disadvantage your own trainees.

Producing the reference
To write an effective reference, you must know about the candidate. Obtain an up-to-date copy of their CV. List what they have achieved during their time in your department. Review information from assessments, discuss their progress with clinical and support staff with whom they work regularly, and check their attendance records if you have access to them.

A typical reference can contain:

- An introduction describing how long you have worked with the applicant
- An assessment of their clinical skills
- A description of their ability to work under pressure
- Recent academic or research successes
- An assessment of the candidates interpersonal skills
- A review of their strengths and weaknesses
- A comment on their attendance record
- A summary of your views of the candidate

Your reference should not duplicate factual information contained in the CV or job application form, it should instead provide the interview committee with additional background information. Examples of the type of comment that might prove valuable to an appointments committee include:

'Though four authors appear on the research paper, the original ideas were all Dr W's.'
'Dr X gets very nervous during interviews and does not perform as well as she might in this setting, although we are quite satisfied that she copes satisfactorily when dealing with clinical emergencies.'
'Dr Y failed to pass his membership examination, but his child was seriously ill just before the examination and he was unable to study as much as he would have liked to have done. I believe that he is making satisfactory academic progress and expect him to pass at the next sitting.'
'Dr Z is a brilliant maverick with no dress sense!'

Bear in mind that some comments virtually preclude a candidate from being appointed. For instance, a sarcastic comment such as 'This doctor's confident manner in no way reflects his clinical skills' is nowadays unwise, and if you write any adverse comments you should be able to justify them on the basis of contemporary written comments made by your senior colleagues and reinforced by reports from formal assessment meetings. If you could not justify your comments to a job tribunal, either change your assessment system, refuse to give references, or give neutral and bland references. The reference that you write forms part of the appointments documentation and an unsuccessful candidate could cite this in evidence if he feels that any part of the appointments procedure has been unfair and wishes to take the case to an industrial tribunal.

Most doctors have a good attendance record. You may wish to comment upon frequent absences, though the information you offer should not breach medical confidentiality. An employing authority can seek further information, if required, through its occupational health physician. If you have access to the information, it is often safer to simply list the number of days absent over the previous 6 months.

A few doctors write dishonest references — supporting a bad candidate to get rid of them from a department, or damning a capable trainee because of a personality clash. This can be done only occasionally as panels become aware of unreliable referees. If a candidates performance at interview is at variance with one of their references, the chairman of the appointments panel ought to tell them that they do not have the support of their referee.

Until recently references were confidential documents which the job applicant did not read. Nowadays the reference is open to legal scrutiny. Some doctors give 'open' references and the trainee receives a copy. References, particularly for consultant posts, used to be supplemented by telephone calls offering confidential background information. Though such calls are still common, under equal opportunities legislation the information they contain can no longer be presented to the interview committee or form part of the official appointments process.

Writing references can be time-consuming and offers no material reward, but it is a pleasure to see your trainees succeed and move up the professional ladder.

Private practice

The main commodity of business is time. Private patients pay for treatment so that they can see more of the specialist, be treated in comfortable surroundings at a time of their choosing, and have adequate privacy, entertainment and communication facilities. The quality of the medical treatment they receive is unlikely to be importantly different from that in the NHS.

General points

Private practice is time-consuming and, for most specialties, involves expensive overheads. Practitioners must to be available whenever they are treating patients. The usual full-time NHS contract allows consultants to earn up to 10% of their income from private practice, but if this 10% limit is exceeded for 2 years, they must transfer to a maximum part-time contract. They then lose one-eleventh of their salary, but retain their fixed clinical commitments. Some trusts offer alternative, more attractive contracts, but these may have other drawbacks so study the fine print carefully. Find out whether there is a group practice in your speciality in your area and, if this method of working appeals to you, ask about the conditions of joining. Many NHS hospitals now have a private wing and practising within this setting means that you will have to travel less.

Private hospitals

The standard of private hospitals has risen substantially in recent years. Most now have resident medical staff, skilled nurses and a high dependency or intensive care unit. Initial contacts will usually be by arranging to meet the hospital manager and matron. Discuss your clinical and administrative requirements to discover whether they can be met. The hospital will want to know how to contact you and you will need a cell phone or pager. Private hospitals are profit-making organizations and will be reluctant to invest in new equipment unless they can get an adequate return on outlay. Some private hospitals seek referrals directly from fund-holding GPs and you must be clear under what terms you would treat these referrals. Fixed price treatment schemes are also common; these save you the effort of billing patients, but the fees paid to you may be lower than you would usually charge. Discover how to book a patient into the hospital and find out if you are expected to follow a particular clinical care pathway.

Marketing

A GMC booklet titled 'Advertising' gives guidance on advertising and publicity. You are entitled to inform local hospitals and GPs that you will accept private patients, and you may advertise providing that you conform to the GMC rules. In private practice you will be a competitor rather than a colleague to other doctors in your speciality. Relations will become strained if you claim a special expertise in a field which they also regard as within their clinical capabilities. It is cynically stated that your success in private practice will depend upon the three 'A's: affability, availability and ability.

Finance

An effective billing and accounting system saves money. Professional help is desirable and your colleagues may know a local accountant who specializes in doctors' financial affairs. Big corporate accountancy companies have big overheads and sometimes charge fees disproportionate to the help they offer an individual. Get expert advice on keeping your books, borrowing money, arranging your finance and savings in a cost effective manner and submitting your tax returns. When you change to a part-time contract, your NHS pension contributions, and therefore your final pension, will drop and you must consider establishing a private pension scheme. Ensure that you have sufficient medical indemnity.

Necessary initial financial procedures include:

- Registering your business with the Inland Revenue. The date that you choose as your financial year-end will affect your cash flow during the first few years you practice
- Arranging a private practice bank account. Banks offer loans to cover initial business expenses before you begin to get income from treating patients. Business rates differ from personal loans
- Arranging medical sickness insurance so that a period of sickness does not result in too drastic a drop in family income
- Reviewing your pension arrangements
- Ensuring that you put enough money aside to pay tax. Your tax bill will arrive over a year after you pay money into your bank account. Do not spend it all meanwhile

Secretary

A good secretary is worth a good salary. Apart from typing your correspondence, a secretary will relieve you of much routine work, such as arranging appointments and admissions. If you have both an NHS and a private practice secretary ensure each knows which part of your life they are organizing, and try to keep a common diary.

Professional people are often reluctant to discuss money with their clients, but your secretary can ensure that your patients have suitable medical insurance or are aware of all the costs that they will incur. Some patients will be insured by their employers, some will have personal insurance and some will be paying their own way. Most will have no idea of the high cost of health care.

Out-patients

Decide when and where you see patients. There are three basic choices:

At home

If your home is suitable, you may wish to establish your practice at home. This decision has considerable implications for your tax position; make sure you understand the implications. You will need to buy medical examination equipment and ensure that you have appropriate secretarial and nursing help. It can be convenient to work from home, but it is expensive initially.

In rooms

In many towns, groups of consultants have clubbed together to purchase a set of consulting rooms. There are benefits in owning a building that may increase in value. Equipment, secretarial and nursing help is shared and can be cheaper. You may be able to buy into one of these sets of rooms, or rent space and help in them.

Working from a private hospital

Renting space in the out-patients department of a private hospital can be the easiest option to start with, as equipment and secretarial help will be provided and diagnostic tools such as X-ray, ultrasound and laboratories may be available. It comes at a price. You may be expected to buy a time-slot which you pay for whether or not you have any patients to see.

The patients

Private patients come from all walks of life and many nations. They are paying for their treatment and expect to receive good quality care on arrangements made by mutual negotiation. They expect to see you regularly. A few may be particularly demanding, but the proportion of them is no higher than within health service practice.

Insurance companies

At the time of writing, the position is that any consultant may treat a patient privately and that the contract for treatment and payment is solely between the doctor and the patient. Doctors may charge any fee they like, although the patient should obviously have an opportunity to agree to or decline both the fee and the treatment. Most insurance companies will reimburse doctors for treating patients insured with them only up to certain limits, and it is essential to inform a patient beforehand if there will be an additional bill to make up a shortfall in insurance payments. Obtain a reimbursement schedule from one of the big insurance companies. Several British insurance companies are attempting to move towards the American Health Maintenance Organization model by trying to limit the number of consultants that they deal with and making them agree to certain agreed treatment plans and re-imbursements. Relations between consultants and some companies have become strained and a newly appointed consultant should consult experienced colleagues before signing any agreements with these companies.

Procedures

Before undertaking a new procedure in a private hospital ensure that you have checked all the equipment that you will require. The theatre staff will be competent, but are unlikely to have specialist knowledge of complex surgical or medical equipment unless they perform the procedure regularly. The hospital probably has arrangements to borrow specialist instruments from another hospital. Ensure all the gear and accessories you need are present before you start. Many operations have been delayed because the light lead for an endoscope has the wrong fitting, or a particular catheter is not available. You are responsible for the equipment you use and should therefore know how to fit things together and be able to cope if some item is not working properly. You cannot so easily overcome a problem by bellowing down the telephone to the clinical engineering department.

Overall

There are two common reasons for doing private practice. The first is to make money, and the second is to enable you to spend some time working to the standards that you would like to achieve, without the constraints imposed by the pressures of the NHS. Although it is still uncommon, some doctors go into full-time private practice because they wish to escape from the managerial confines of the NHS. Before committing yourself to a time-consuming enterprise, which will substantially reduce the time you have spare for leisure and your family, ensure you know what your motives are.

Further reading

The British Medical Association publishes *The Consultants' Handbook*, which gives detailed information about contracts and terms of service for senior hospital staff. The third edition was published in 1997 and can be obtained by BMA members from BMA House, Tavistock Square, London WC1H 9JP.

BUPA, the medical insurance company, produce *A Guide to Private Consultant Practice*. This was updated in 1997, and is available from: The Medical Communications Team, BUPA, 15–19 Bloomsbury Way, London WC1A 2BA.

12. THE STRUCTURE OF HEALTH CARE

Objectives of this section
- to understand how health care is paid for
- to know who are 'purchasers' and 'providers'
- to realize why it is difficult to price the cost of a treatment
- to understand the problems of doctors in management

Health care systems worldwide have serious organizational and financial problems. In developed countries, new technology and the demands of an ageing population mean that the cost of care is rising inexorably; in the developing world, economic crises and high birth rates mean that even basic health care is an unaffordable luxury. As a consultant you are responsible for initiating expensive treatments and must understand their financial implications.

Historical perspective

People have always tried to care for the sick. Infirmaries and poor houses existed in ancient civilizations. Initially many sick houses were attached to religious foundations and the tradition of linking spiritual and physical well-being continued until the 18th century when civil authorities started to build municipal hospitals. In the 19th century, the discovery of anaesthesia and asepsis allowed complex surgery to develop, but more expensive facilities and better trained staff were needed. The early 20th century saw the introduction of radiology and the beginnings of the pharmaceutical industry. Most hospitals remained funded by a mixture of patient fees and charitable donations until the second world war, when medical technology accelerated and the cost of a chronic illness or major operation outstripped the ability of individuals to pay for their treatment.

Politicians tackled this problem in a variety of ways. Some, believing that health care is a fundamental human right, sought to offer access to health care equally to their whole population regardless of wealth; others deliberately, or simply by default, established systems that favoured the rich. Box 12.1 shows four models of funding health.

Social funds, compulsory national systems of insurance, are common in continental Europe. Hospitals and individual doctors bill these funds and receive payment for services. Social funds have found it difficult to control medical expenditure and many are now in financial difficulty, a situation made worse by an excess of doctors in some countries.

Box 12.1. Methods of paying for health care

Socialized medicine	Britain, Sweden	State-funded, salary or capitation fees	Everyone covered
Socialized insurance	Canada, France	Single payer, fee-for-service	Everyone covered
Mandatory insurance	Germany, Japan	Multiple sickness funds, salaried staff or fee-for-service	Everyone covered
Voluntary insurance	USA, South Africa	Multiple systems of payment	No universal cover

Other countries rely on commercial *insurance companies* to fund health care. The insurance organization may be a quasi-autonomous non-governmental organization (quango) or a commercial company. Individuals, or more commonly their employers, pay premiums to the insurance company which then pays the bills after an illness. There is usually some safety-net to protect the unemployed and chronically sick.

In the USA the purely commercially driven system of independent hospitals and private physicians resulted in high-costs and inequality of provision. Insurance companies tried to control costs by a variety of auditing mechanisms, but failed. Premiums rose constantly to cover the escalating costs, but major companies became alarmed by the high premiums demanded for covering their staff. They turned instead to *Health Maintenance Organizations*. HMOs are commercial companies which contract to look after all the health needs of their client groups. They provide a comprehensive service, owning clinics and hospitals, and employing staff. Some have become very powerful and demand that patients covered by their schemes receive care only according to their approved *managed-care* pathways. The HMOs have at last stabilized the cost of health care in the USA, forcing inefficient hospitals to close and driving down medical remuneration. Medical insurers in other parts of the world are considering following this system. However, there is concern that the mandatory managed-care pathways sometimes favour economy over quality. Unless doctors are prepared to assess the care they offer and control their own budgets, someone else will do it for them and that is likely to be unwelcome.

Organization of health care in Britain

In Britain groups of *primary care clinicians* (GPs, nurses, midwives and health visitors) provide community care and act as gatekeepers for specialist facilities. Most specialist facilities are provided in *district general hospitals* (DGH) each serving a local population of about 300,000. Patients may be referred from the DGH to tertiary referral centres serving populations of about two million for highly specialized treatments such as cardiac and neurosurgery. The gatekeeper function of the primary care clinicians successfully limits access to expensive hospital facilities and is being copied elsewhere. There is debate about whether the DGH will remain the appropriate place for the delivery of specialist care in the 21st century. One argument is that many treatments such as day-case surgery should be provided at *community hospitals* or *polyclinics* near to the patients, while specialized services should be centred on a few big high-technology hospitals serving populations of about two million.

Many countries have never developed the British system of primary care physicians. Instead, patients themselves select a specialist who makes arrangements for treatment in the local clinic or referral to a major hospital. The patient is able to select from a wider choice of specialists, but must themselves select the correct specialty for their underlying problem.

Funding health care in Britain

The British socialized system means that the government, through taxation, is responsible for paying for health care. Central control has resulted in cost-effective medicine with one of the lowest expenditures per person in the developed world, but has restricted access to expensive treatments. A smaller proportion of gross national product is spent on health care in Britain than in most developed countries.

From the establishment of the NHS in 1945 until the 1989 reform, the government was directly responsible for funding the health service. This system was cheap and simple to run. Its disadvantage was that a complex bureaucracy developed with decisions based more on political priorities than on local need. It was perceived to be cumbersome and inflexible, with funding based upon historic allocations to individual units, rather than the ability of those units to deliver cost-effective health care. The system became a political liability as the government was perceived to be responsible for all failures in the service. The 1989 reform distanced government from operational matters. A system of competing *purchasers* and *providers* was established (Box 12.2). The Treasury simply transferred an annual allocation to the NHS executive, a quasi-business organization, which in turn became responsible for distributing money to the purchasers of health care and regulating the providers.

Purchasers are given money according to a 'per capita' funding formula to pay for the health care of their population. Government-funded purchasers include *district health authorities*, *consortia* of GPs, or individual *fund-holding general practices*. Although they are not funded by government, medical

---

Box 12.2. Purchasers and providers in the British health system

Purchasers	Providers
Local District Health Authorities	Hospitals (NHS and Private sector)
Other health authorities (extra-contractual referrals, ECRs)	Community and Mental Health Trusts
GP fundholders	Ambulance Trusts
GP consortia	GPs
NHS Executive (ring-fenced funds)	Other practitioners
Private insurance companies	(Physio/chiropractors)
Universities (education and research)	
Research councils (MRC)	
Pharmaceutical companies	
Charities	

---

insurance companies are also purchasers of health care, and a variety of other organizations such as *charities* and *universities* may buy specific treatments or elements of education. The purchaser can, in theory, choose how to spend their funds for the benefit of their patients and are free to shop around the various provider organizations.

The Conservative government in the early 1990s encouraged the development of GP fundholding schemes. The initial fundholding practices purchased a limited range of elective procedures from hospitals together with some support services such as physiotherapy and radiology. Total fundholding then developed. With total control over their budget, the GP gatekeeper becomes the point of rationing of healthcare resources. As long as their funds are adequate, GPs welcome the flexibility and power that comes from controlling their own budgets; but some practices consume more resources than others and those forced to make difficult decisions about which treatments to fund may lose their initial enthusiasm. Purchasing consortia of group practices may eventually prove an effective compromise between the various systems, enabling GPs to advocate the care they want for their communities, without requiring them to deal with too many day-to-day financial problems.

Providers are individuals, clinics or organizations that treat patients during an acute illness or that offer long-term care. They consume resources. Providers in the British NHS are quangos. They are structured as businesses, but their activities are controlled far more rigidly than profit-making businesses. For instance, they are obliged to charge only what it costs to treat a patient, and legislation governs where and how they may raise funds for developments. They have very tight financial controls and their budgets at the end of the year should be within 0.5% of their targets. Managers of an

NHS Trust have the difficult task of balancing many conflicting demands and a good senior manager deserves the sympathy rather than the scorn of clinicians. Other organizations such as private hospitals, hospices and charitable institutions can also contract to provide care. In the early period after the reforms, competition was encouraged, but it then became apparent that it was not beneficial or cost-effective to have many small units all offering similar services. Political dogma is moving back from encouraging competition to favouring co-operation.

Contracts

Purchaser/provider contracts specify the type of health care to be provided. The original aim of the reforms was to 'make money follow patients' and to reward efficient units. This aim has not been realized. Most contracts still conform to the *block contract* model. In this model, the provider agrees to provide health care for a group of conditions (for example, obstetric services or acute medical conditions) for a particular annual sum of money. Block contracts are easy to manage and ensure that a trust has a fixed income to cover its running expenses. However, if workload increases unpredictably and expensively, the trust cannot increase its income and has to find the money to treat the additional patients from its own reserves. Block contracts are crude and inflexible. They may simply specify that a certain number of in-patient cases must be treated and this rigidity can prevent clinicians introducing cheaper out-patient treatments. In general, purchasers favour block contracts, but providers are becoming progressively disillusioned with them.

Fee-for-service contracts enable trusts to charge an appropriate fee for a treatment, but running such contracts is expensive as the cost of each treatment must be analysed and an invoice produced for each patient. Furthermore, fee-for-service contracts may encourage providers to undertake unnecessary investigations. The flexibility of these contracts permits quicker variations in patient referral patterns and so offers improved freedom of choice and higher standards of care for the patients, but this freedom can create problems for providers as it takes many years to build up expertise in a particular specialist field, while a transient lack of funding can rapidly destroy a unit. This dilemma is unresolved, although it has been suggested that long-term contracts will have to be established between providers and purchasers to ensure that specialist units survive.

Costing a hospital admission

Superficially it might seem simple to cost a hospital admission; in practice it is difficult. Hospitals are complex labour-intensive organizations. The hospital must pay not only clinicians such as doctors, nurses and physiotherapists, but must also provide support staff such as laboratory staff, porters and secretaries, as well as a large group of people not involved in directly caring for patients such as managers, engineers, technicians and gardeners. Salaries make up two-thirds of all running costs. The other third of the costs of the organization are concerned with maintaining and heating the buildings and paying for purchase and maintenance of equipment. There is no common formula for distributing these costs between in-patients and out-patients, between out-of-hours emergency patients and elective admissions, or between people staying a long time and short admissions. Because individual hospitals distribute these costs in different ways, the charges that they make for performing similar procedures can vary enormously. The efficiency of hospitals also varies, but is equally difficult to quantify.

Management structure and finance in trusts

An NHS Trust receives the funds its needs from the purchasers listed in Box 12.2. These include:

- Contracts with purchasing authorities and GPs
- Fees from insurance companies for looking after private patients
- Charitable funding of specific staff or research projects
- University funding of staff to enable teaching and research to be performed

In addition larger hospitals will receive money from referrals from one consultant to another with highly specialized skills — a system known as extra-contractual referrals.

Finally certain initiatives may be paid for centrally by the NHS Executive who transfer money for a specific purpose, so called *ring-fenced funds*. The development of clinical audit and hospital sign-posting schemes were paid for by ring-fenced money. The amalgamation of these funds produces the annual hospital budget, which must be divided between the various services in the hospital.

The Trust Board is responsible for control of the whole organization. It is a quango whose constitution is controlled by law. The Trust Board includes both executive and non-executive directors. The executive directors typically include the chief executive, the finance director, the medical director of the hospital and another representative clinician. The non-executive directors are appointed by the Secretary of State for Health and are prominent members of the local community brought in to provide outside expertise and different perspectives on health care. The chair of the trust is one of the non-executive directors and is the public figurehead of the organization. Chairmen have interpreted their roles in a variety of ways and some have been highly controversial; however, the real power and responsibility lies with the chief executive who has the final authority to sign contracts and approve expenditure. Conflict between these two powerful figures is an organizational disaster, as indeed are any major splits on the Trust Board.

Below board level the organization of trusts varies. Some are management-led with the budgets being controlled by full-time managers, who seek advice from clinicians in making their decisions. Other trusts are led by clinicians with an important Clinical Management Board making decisions about how the trust should develop. The clinical directors of the various departments in the hospital hold their own budgets, supported by management and administrative staff. The clinical director is responsible for recruiting staff, providing a service, ensuring that training is effective, encouraging innovation and is professionally responsible for the quality of the service that the directorate offers.

There is a fundamental conflict when doctors become involved in management. Doctors are trained to look after the health of the patient in front of them regardless of the implications of their actions to society as a whole. For instance, the cost of blood given to the trauma victim is not seen as a consideration that the operating team should take into account when dealing with the results of a road accident. Clinical directors have to cope with a different problem. They are given a finite budget and told that they must not overspend. They must therefore manage their units in such a way that the greatest good is done to the greatest number of patients. Management is about compromise but this can lead to conflict if clinicians believe that departmental management policies designed to control cost are preventing optimum care being given to individual patients.

On the one hand, the number of clinicians willing to participate in management is small, and the rewards are limited. On the other hand, doctors have a choice — either they manage themselves or they are managed by others. The second alternative is usually perceived to be less desirable.

The underlying dilemma of health care

By 1990, the cost of medical advances exceeded the ability of any country to afford the highest technology care for all its population. Taxpayers and those paying insurance premiums refused to accept further price rises. Audit revealed that there was little correlation between the amount of money poured into acute health services and the general health of the population served. Politicians and insurers do not like to be seen to be 'rationing' health care and have tried to improve the cost-effectiveness of health services under their control by improving the 'efficiency' of services with the aim that all hospitals should match the standards of care of the most efficient. Creating financial savings by this process has been a controversial process and is the basis of many of the tensions in health care today.

In developed countries there are now more dependent elderly people consuming resources and proportionally fewer people in productive jobs producing wealth. From a purely economic viewpoint, and excluding any moral dimension, a medical intervention is only effective if the patient returns to productive work themselves; or needs less care, so freeing someone else to work. A treatment that prolongs life without reducing dependence costs money but has no economic benefit. Even effective treatments such as thrombolytic treatment for myocardial infarction add to the overall cost of health care, as the patient might not die (cheaply!) during the initial episode, but instead survive and require further expensive therapies to prolong life, before ultimately dying. After all, everyone dies in the end. About two-thirds of the healthcare resources that an individual consumes are required during the last 6 months of life; the trouble is that one cannot predict which 6 months it will be until afterwards.

The growing gap between what is possible and what is affordable means that people often realize that they, or their relatives, are not receiving the best possible care. As a result health systems are perceived to be failing.

The health of the population

Most hospitals treat acute illness. This is expensive, and affects the overall health of the population far less than unglamorous public health measures such as sanitation and immunization. Inequalities in society such as poverty and unemployment also affect health. Box 12.3 lists some of the important factors that control the health of whole communities. Governments have the power to influence people in these fields, the caring professions by themselves are nearly impotent. British government initiatives such as the *Health of the Nation* were designed to re-focus the attention of professionals from the glamorous high-tech achievements of acute care, many of which only benefit a handful of very ill patients, towards less exciting but more generally beneficial public health measures.

Box 12.3. Factors affecting the health of populations

- Access to primary care
- Water fluoridation
- Diet
- Life-style
- Obesity
- Education
- Employment
- Wealth
- Social deprivation
- Smoking
- Transport
- Pollution
- Sanitation
- Geographical variations

---

13. SOCIETY, MEDICINE AND DOCTORS

Objectives of this section

- to understand the role of doctors in society
- to understand how and why medical ethics have changed
- to provide a framework for ethical decision making

'Priests see people at their best, lawyers at their worst, but doctors see them as they really are'. Doctors are unique in their involvement in major life events — birth, sickness, death, — and deal with people during their most vulnerable moments. They are allowed unparalleled access; people bare themselves physically and mentally in intimate detail. This level of trust is an extraordinary privilege, and being worthy of it is a tremendous responsibility. But trust is not automatic, it needs to be earned, and once earned, maintained. Doctors can only work within the context of the society in which they live, and must adapt as society changes. Medicine is driven by internal and external forces which constantly redefine what doctors can do, and equally importantly, how they are perceived.

Amongst the forces affecting medicine are technological change, social structures and political imperatives. These forces have complex interactions. For instance fibre-optic technology has revolutionized surgery, permitting minimally invasive approaches to some surgical problems and allowing short-stay surgery. Doctors have had to learn radically different technical skills, but patients have seen advantages in that they now prefer, whenever possible, to be cared for at home rather than staying in hospital. Society at large benefits from the cheaper hospital care and money can be spent elsewhere.

Political change affects how doctors work: the Patient's Charter, the purchaser–provider split, and GP fundholding have all altered expectations of how health care is delivered. The Calman report, driven by European legislation, has resulted in the introduction of structured specialist training very different from the previous apprenticeship system, and is making very different demands on trainers and trainees. Medicine has embraced the media; we are positively bombarded with information about health, disease and medical practice, sometimes accurate and useful, often sadly, wrong and harmful.

These changes affect the public perception of doctors and the way that doctors see themselves. This section looks at the role of the doctor, focuses on some of the ethical issues that are changing medical practice and finally suggests an approach to the most challenging problems in medicine, which are not technical or clinical but humanitarian. As Richard Smith, editor of the

BMJ wrote in an editorial in March 1997 titled 'All doctors are problem doctors':

> Doctors are set apart. We are a priesthood with our own rites, beliefs, systems of initiation and tribal practices. And we have special powers. The public turns to us in moments of extremity and expects an answer, even a solution. Often we cannot provide it. We cannot defeat death, sickness and pain. Everybody within the priesthood knows its vulnerability. But the public doesn't know about that vulnerability. They hope we can deliver and we want to. Indeed our privileges depend upon being able to. We are thus permanently conflicted: expected and wanting to deliver but not often able to.

The doctor is a unique amalgam, the nature of whose composition has always provoked thought — father figure or plumber, engineer or priest suggest a range of roles not seen in other occupations. It is worth a brief look at the development of the modern doctor to help understand the roots of these attitudes.

The historical context

The *Medical Act* of 1858 and its amendment in 1886 established for the first time a register of qualified doctors. Before this time individuals who called themselves doctor and practised a form of medicine might not have had any kind of qualification at all. With no recognized system that produced doctors, a variety of people involved themselves in 'healing', from the gentleman who had acquired some knowledge and practised as a hobby with no pecuniary gain, to the 'quack' who sold usually ineffective and occasionally dangerous patent medicines to a gullible public. (The name 'quack' derives either from 'quack salber' — quicksilver or mercury used to treat venereal disease, or from the practice of 'quacking' wares at open air markets.) Some doctors were qualified, possessing degrees, licenses or diplomas from a variety — as many as 18 — institutions of variable respectability. Some of the qualifications were purely local, conveying the right to practice in one city, but not elsewhere.

The *Medical Act* of 1858 came into being in part because of public pressure for a system that would allow reputable practitioners to be identified, but also following pressure from the Colleges of Physicians and Surgeons, and the Society of Apothecaries to exert influence on and wield power over the development of medicine and medical education. Their success in framing the legislation enhanced the status of the three institutions and meant that the roles of physician, surgeon and apothecary, up to that time easily identifiable, began to merge, eventually producing the modern doctor.

Physicians considered themselves to be at the top of the pecking order, and certainly had higher status. They would usually have attended a university, undertaking the broadly based classical education that was the norm for the gentleman of the day. Clinical experience was obtained by apprenticeship to a practising physician for an unspecified period of time, observing cases and learning methods. Practice was based almost exclusively on detailed history taking, physical examination being perfunctory, if performed at all. Indeed, cases could be, and often were, managed on the basis of an exchange of letters. This rather lofty detachment served to reinforce the physicians status; gentleman by birth, scholar by education, a member of a learned profession.

Surgeons, on the other hand, had much humbler origins, not losing their association with Barbers until 1745, with the establishment of the Company of Surgeons. Surgical skills were acquired purely by apprenticeship, without a preceding general education. They tended to be middle rather than upper class and their association with pain and suffering in the pre-anaesthetic era made them feared as well as respected. Speedy surgery was matter of great pride. Robert Liston, regarded as the most dextrous 19th century surgeon, before beginning an amputation would ask watching students to 'Time me gentlemen, time me'. The surgeon required: 'the eye of an eagle, the strength of a giant and the hand of a lady', as well as the fortitude needed to inflict appalling pain.

Apothecaries were shopkeepers, originally grocers, who made and sold medicines — 'pill-pushers'. They were supposed only to dispense what the physician prescribed and not to engage in diagnosis, but, in rural areas where there were fewer physicians, they began to see patients themselves, adding diagnosis and prescribing to the dispensing role. They were in this way the forerunner of the GP, and only referred the more complicated cases to surgeons and physicians. Pharmacists are still approached for medical advice, and often give it, quite properly and legally as anyone can practice medicine in the UK, unlike the care of animals where it is illegal for anyone but a qualified vet to prescribe and treat.

The newly regulated and registered medical profession created a system of medical education, whose content was strictly controlled by the Society of Apothecaries and the Colleges. Anything disapproved of was excluded, and contact with what we now call 'alternative practitioners' was not considered proper, and even subject to the ultimate sanction, suspension or erasure from the medical register. It is only within the last 10–15 years that this rigid attitude has relaxed; a more 'holistic' approach now obtains, and osteopathy, chiropractic and acupuncture have achieved a measure of acceptance and respectability.

Medicine — trade or profession

Implicit to the role of the doctor throughout has been an underlying set of ethics; society has to believe that doctors are guided by a set of underlying principles that regulate what they can and should do. Doctors are plumbers, they are technicians; they ply a trade for which they are paid. But they are more than that. For their own benefit, and that of society, doctors need to be able to answer the question: 'what is a doctor?'.

Oaths, codes and declarations

A profession differs from a trade in that it incorporates a code of behaviour. This code forms the basis on which the profession regulates itself. Self-regulation is a privilege, awarded to a profession by society for as long as that profession remains sensitive to changing attitudes in society. Codes and oaths are a public expression of a profession's contract with society. The medical profession has had a code of practice — originally enshrined in the Hippocratic Oath — for nearly three millennia. An examination of the various professional oaths shows how the role of the doctor has changed over time.

Although certain injunctions regarding the duties of doctors appear in the Code of Laws of the Babylonian king Hammurabi dated 1790 BC, the oath attributed to the School of Hippocrates, the Greek physician born on the island of Kos in about 460 BC, is regarded as the archetypal medical behav-

---

Box 13.1. The Hippocratic Oath

I swear by Apollo the physician, by Aesculapus, by Hygieia, by Panacea, and by all the gods and goddesses making them my witnesses, that I will carry out according to my ability and judgement this oath and this indenture. To hold my teacher in this art equal to my own parents; to make him partner in my livelihood; when he is in need of money to share mine with him; to consider his family as my own brothers, and to teach them this art, if they want to learn it, without fee or indenture; to impart precept, oral instruction and all other instruction to my own sons, the sons of my teacher, and to pupils who have taken the physicians oath, but to nobody else.

I will follow that system of regimen which, according to my ability and judgement, I consider for the benefit of my patients, and abstain from whatever is deleterious and mischievous. I will give no deadly medicine to anyone if asked, nor suggest any such counsel; and in like manner I will not give to a woman a pessary to produce abortion. With purity and with holiness I will pass my life and practice my Art. I will not cut persons labouring under the stone, but will leave this to be done by men who are practitioners of this work. Into whatever houses I enter, I will go into them for the benefit of the sick, and will abstain from every voluntary act of mischief and corruption; and further, from the seduction of females, or males, or freemen or slaves. Whatever in connection with my professional practice, not in connection with it, I see or hear, in the life of men, which ought not to be spoken of abroad, I will not divulge, as reckoning that all such should be kept secret.

While I continue to keep this Oath unviolated, may it be granted to me to enjoy life and the practice of the Art, respected by all men, in all times. But should I trespass and violate this Oath, may the reverse be my lot.

---

iour code. It is worth quoting in one of its many English translations and comparing it with subsequent attempts to bring it up to date (Box 13.1).

The oath is in four parts:

The preamble: 'I swear to Apollo...' invokes the supernatural and emphasizes the sacred nature of the calling. In today's secular society allusions to religion would be out of place.

The covenant: 'To hold my teacher...' This makes it clear that the oath taker is joining a select group whose members look after each other and keep their special knowledge to themselves. Now doctors are encouraged to promote awareness of health and disease and disseminate as much information as possible.

The code: 'I will use treatment...' The code defines the boundaries of the 'doctor–patient relationship, mainly in terms of what should not be done — do not (intentionally) do harm, do not use the doctor's privileged position for personal gain of any kind.

The peroration: 'Now if I carry out this oath...' The doctor must stick to the rules; breaking any of them will result in expulsion from the group, with its attendant loss of position, authority and status. The modern doctor needs to be aware of contemporary standards, who sets them and the procedures that can follow failure to maintain them.

In 1947, the newly formed World Medical Association restated the Hippocratic Oath in modern language (Box 13.2). It was prompted to do so because of the involvement of doctors in the so-called 'medical experiments' carried out by the Nazis during the second world war. It reads (as amended in 1983):

Box 13.2. The Declaration of Geneva (1947)

At the time of being admitted as a member of the Medical Profession: I solemnly pledge myself to consecrate my life to the service of humanity; I will give my teachers the respect and gratitude which is their due; I will practice my profession with conscience and dignity; The health of my patient will be my first consideration; I will respect the secrets which are confided in me, even after the patient has died; I will maintain by all the means in my power, the honour and the noble traditions of the medical profession; My colleagues will be my brothers; I will not permit considerations of religion, nationality, race, party politics or social standing to intervene between my duty and my patients; I will maintain the utmost respect for human life from its beginning even under threat and I will not use my medical knowledge contrary to the laws of humanity; I make these promises solemnly, freely and upon my honour.

The Declaration has, of course, been overtaken by events. The *Abortion Act* of 1967 made termination of pregnancy legal up to 28 weeks (now amended to 24 weeks except to prevent grave permanent injury to the physical or mental health of the woman, to reduce the risk to her life, or if there is a risk that the foetus would suffer from such physical or mental abnormalities as to be seriously handicapped after birth). This is clearly incompatible with the injunction to 'maintain the utmost respect for human life from its beginning...'.

In recognition of this and other ethical issues, the BMA issued in 1997, 50 years after the *Declaration of Geneva*, a revised oath (Box 13.3). It received a mixed press to say the least; both its content and the need for a revision at all were questioned. A poet has been hired to make its language more mellifluous. It does though reflect the attitudes of part of the medical establishment and is worth comparing with its predecessors.

Much of the BMA oath makes explicit what is implicit in the original, but there are differences. Responsibility within society and not just to individual patients is alluded to; for instance confidentiality is made conditional: 'overriding reasons' can allow a doctor to disclose information about a patient if it is in the public interest. Abortion is acknowledged to be part of medicine if performed ethically. But probably the most radical change occurs in the sentence 'I recognize the special value of human life, but I also know that the prolongation of human life is not the only aim of health care'. It is probably quite deliberate that this statement is not analysed in more detail, for it involves issues and situations presented to doctors that are often the most troubling and difficult to deal with.

A simple problem, say a hernia, has a simple solution — an operation with low morbidity and high efficacy. But some problems are more difficult, and can provoke much soul-searching. They lie for the most part in the 'grey areas' of medicine. They have little to do with clinical knowledge or technical skills. They concern the appropriateness of care. Should a treatment be offered to a patient? How long should it continue? When should it be stopped? How do you decide? These issues are amongst the most taxing problems doctors face. We can do many things to and for patients: choosing the right thing is the problem.

Until recently, doctors were paternalistic and authoritarian. Patients were told what they needed (doctor's orders) and accepted passively (you're the doctor). When the patient became a 'client', however, the relationship underwent subtle changes. The client comes to the doctor to accept or reject all or part of the proffered advice. The client has ownership of his health (and disease) and wishes to be an active participant in the decision making process. The skill to analyse clinical and ethical problems and communicate

Box 13.3. The British Medical Association Oath (1997)

The practice of medicine is a privilege which carries important responsibilities. All doctors should observe the core values of the profession, which centre on the duty to help sick people and avoid harm. I promise that my medical knowledge will be used to benefit people's health. They are my first concern. I will listen to them and provide the best care I can. I will be honest, respectful and compassionate towards the patients.

In emergencies, I will do my best to help anyone in medical need. I will make every effort to ensure that the rights of all patients are respected including vulnerable groups who lack means of making their needs known, be it through immaturity, mental incapacity, imprisonment or detention or other circumstances.

My professional judgement will be exercised as independently as possible and not be influenced by political pressure nor by factors such as social standing of the patient.

I will not put personal profit or advancement above my duty to patients. I recognise the special value of human life but I also know that the prolongation of human life is not the only aim of health care. Where abortion is permitted, I agree that it should take place only within an ethical and legal framework. I will not provide treatments which are pointless or harmful or which an informed and competent patient refuses.

I will ensure patients receive the information and support they want to make decisions about disease prevention and improvement of their health.

I will answer as truthfully as I can and respect patients' decisions unless that puts others at risk of harm. If I cannot agree with their requests, I will explain why. If my patients have limited mental awareness I will still encourage them to participate in decisions as much as they feel able and willing to do so.

I will maintain confidentiality about all patients. If there are overriding reasons which prevent my keeping a patient's confidentiality I will explain them. I will recognise the limits of my knowledge and seek advice from colleagues when necessary. I will acknowledge my mistakes. I will do my best to keep myself and my colleagues informed of new developments and ensure that poor standards or bad practices are exposed to those who can improve them. I will show respect for all those with whom I work and be ready to share my knowledge by teaching others what I know. I will use my training and professional standing to improve the community in which I work. I will treat patients equitably and support fair and human distribution of health resources. I will try to influence positively authorities whose policies harm public health. I will oppose policies which breach internationally accepted standards of human rights. I will strive to change laws which are contrary to patients' interests or my professional ethics

the reasons for decisions is as important as any technical ability. Doctors need to learn a logical approach to decision making that is effective and can bear scrutiny.

An ethical approach to decision making in medicine

Timing is an integral part of decisions about appropriateness of treatments. What is justifiable one day may not be the next. Cases need to be reviewed regularly using the same system and criteria each time.

The 'Four Principles' approach

The four principles of medical ethics are:

- Respect for autonomy
- Beneficence
- Non-maleficence
- Distributive justice

These principles are discussed in more detail in T Beauchamp and J Childress, *Principles of Biomedical Ethics*, 4th Edition. Oxford University Press, Oxford, 1994.

Though important in ethical debate, these principles cannot form the exclusive basis of a universal decision-making process. Using them, however, helps both decision making and communication, and enables doctors to justify their actions.

Respect for autonomy

Autonomy is the freedom of competent individuals to determine their own actions and behaviours. Assessment of competence is an issue in itself, but for the purpose of this discussion it is assumed that the patient has the right to influence his health care and that the doctor should respect that right — 'whose life is it anyway?'

Beneficence

The obligation to act for the benefit of others. In the context of the doctor–patient relationship, actions should be directed towards a good outcome.

Non-maleficence

Closely linked to beneficence is the obligation not to inflict harm intentionally. The Latin legal tag is 'Primum non nocere' — first do no harm.

Distributive justice

Health care should be distributed fairly, appropriately and with equity.

Most of the time the principles can be reconciled. A simple operation that cures a painful or restricting condition, restoring normal activity, albeit at the expense of some postoperative pain (which a doctor would try to minimize) clearly satisfies all four. But when the principles conflict, problems are more difficult to resolve. Under these circumstances the medical profession may not be able to resolve the problem and the law becomes involved. To illustrate the principles in practice, some cases where disagreements about treatment have reached the law courts have been selected.

The Wanglie Case (USA)

Helga Wanglie, aged 86, sustained a cardiac arrest during an admission to hospital for a severe chest infection and chronic bronchiectasis. She was resuscitated, but tests over the next few weeks convinced the medical staff that she was in a persistent vegetative state secondary to brain hypoxia. She was maintained on a ventilator, treated with antibiotics, physiotherapy and enteral nutrition. Several times over the next weeks, it was suggested to her family that the treatment was not benefiting her and should be withdrawn. Their response was 'that physicians should not play God, that removing her life support showed moral decay in our civilization, and that a miracle could occur'. The hospital, after several months of impasse, approached the Florida Supreme Court, initially asking it to appoint an independent conservator who would determine whether continued treatment was beneficial. The intention was that if the conservator agreed that treatment was not beneficial to seek a ruling that it could be discontinued. The court appointed 87- year-old Mr Wanglie as conservator. Three days later, Mrs Wanglie died of septic shock. Her hospitalization had lasted 18 months and cost $700,000. This judgement in favour of autonomy created a precedent. The issues of the likelihood of the care being beneficial and the appropriateness and possible harmful effects of the therapies used could not be raised in the court; Mr Wanglie had already made his views clear and by appointing him conservator the court excluded anything but autonomy from consideration.

Re J (a minor) (child in care: medical treatment)

When 1 month old, J was involved in a road traffic accident, sustaining injuries resulting in microcephaly, cortical blindness, uncontrollable convulsions and severe developmental retardation. Over the ensuing months, J required frequent hospitalization. When aged 1 year, the medical team discussed the withdrawal of active resuscitation with J's mother on the grounds that he would not develop further, had a reduced life expectancy in which distressing painful interventions were required — maleficence without beneficence, harm to no benefit. The mother wanted full active treatment to be continued. When this case eventually reached the Court of Appeal the court ruled that it was not its place to order a medical practitioner to treat a patient contrary to his clinical judgement and perception of duty of care. Patient autonomy, albeit by surrogate, was overruled in favour of beneficence and non-maleficence. In a virtually identical case in the USA, 'baby L', when a judge ascertained that the clinical team would not continue active resuscitation even if so ordered by the court, another hospital was found to take over the child's care. The court appeared therefore to accept all three principles — cost of care had not been an issue.

The case of 'child B'

Child B, a 10-year-old leukaemia sufferer was refused the opportunity of a second bone marrow transplant when her leukaemia relapsed. This was in spite of a clearly expressed wish by the child and her father in favour of undergoing the treatment. Child B, Jaymee Bowen was clearly 'competent' in the legal sense to take this decision; she had been through it before and clearly knew what she was talking about. The doctor in the case made her judgement against a transplant based on its chances of success weighed against the trauma of the chemotherapy, that is on beneficience and non-maleficence; it would not work and would expose the patient to unnecessary pain and suffering. When the father challenged the decision in the High Court, the health authority brought the £75,000 cost of the treatment into the equation, stating broadly the utilitarian view that it was not in the greatest good of the greatest number to allocate this resource in this situation. The court told the authority to reconsider its refusal and the case went to appeal. Judgement in the Court of Appeal was in favour of Cambridge Health Authority. The authority had been right and proper to consider the interests of 'other patients' in allocating resources that were not limitless, in other words, thinking in terms of distributive justice.

Analysing problems using the principles has the virtue of being systematic. It must be done though with compassion, in good faith, and to no personal gain. Balancing autonomy, beneficience and non-maleficence is an integral part of the doctor–patient relationship. Decision making based on weighing them relative to one another can be easily communicated even if the words themselves are not used. Consideration of distributive justice fits less easily, but in a cash-limited health service its existence cannot be denied; prioritization is part of medicine. The decision in the case of child B endorsed the validity of bringing fair allocation of resources into treatment decisions involving individual patients. Doctors cannot escape from the responsibility, as members of society if nothing more, of giving distributive justice a place in the decision-making process — a last place maybe, but there.

This approach, sometimes called, pejoratively 'principalism' has been said to bring a 'cookbook' approach to moral issues that is inappropriate. Be that as it may, in the real clinical world it is helpful to have a structure, if for no other reason than that it demonstrates that decisions are made in a thoughtful, consistent manner.

Doctors, duties, discipline and complaints

One of the hallmarks of a profession is a degree of self-regulation. Doctors are subject to the rule of law like all citizens, but in fulfilling their professional obligations they are expected to conform to standards set, largely, by the profession itself. Until recently these standards were for the most part, implicit — a doctor was, well, a doctor, and society trusted the profession to ensure the integrity of its practitioners, without asking many questions. Things have changed. 'Consumers' have become more demanding, expecting explicit descriptions of the 'goods and services' they are to receive. How 'self-regulation' can affect individual doctors has also changed.

This section looks at the duties of a doctor as seen by the profession's self regulatory body, and how it has affected complaints procedures and discipline.

The GMC

The GMC has as its primary function the maintenance of the medical register, the list of doctors entitled to call themselves 'registered medical practitioners' and without which legal status they could not hold NHS appointments (as doctors), prescribe certain drugs, or sign death and other official certificates. The administration involved in maintaining the register is the largest part of the GMC's work. In addition, it has an important role in the supervision of undergraduate and post-graduate medical education, and is responsible for issuing Certificates of Completion of Specialist Training, following the recommendations of the Calman report.

The composition of the council underlines the extent to which medicine is a self-regulating profession. Since 1978 it has comprised 102 members, of whom 54 are directly elected by postal ballot of all registered medical practitioners in the UK (England 42, Scotland 7, Wales 3, and Northern Ireland 2). There are 21 members nominated by universities with medical faculties, 14 appointed by the Royal Colleges, Faculties and the Society of Apothecaries. Finally 13 members, (11 lay and 2 medical) are appointed by the Queen, on the advice of the Privy Council. Of the 102 members, 91 are doctors. The elected members, if all acted together, could be held to constitute a permanent in-built majority — the medical profession is truly 'self-regulating'.

A small, but high profile, part of the self-regulation has been the disciplinary functions of the GMC, seen most clearly in the work of the 'Professional Conduct Committee. This committee deals with allegations of 'serious professional misconduct' — a definition which includes activities verging on the criminal, which are dealt with in a manner very similar to the judicial system used in civil and criminal law. Doctors appearing before the PCC have been charged as a result of closely defined allegations made by witnesses testifying on oath. However this committee is not allowed to investigate professional incompetence. In a society which now demands explicitness in most aspects of life, work and behaviour, this has become an anomaly, and unsustainable.

Duties of a doctor

In keeping with its perception that there was a need for professional standards to be made more explicit, the GMC issued, in October 1995 the booklet *Duties of a Doctor*, setting out what were described as 'principles of good practice'. The introductory paragraph is reproduced here (Box 13.4).

Box 13.4. Duties of a doctor

Being registered with the General Medical Council gives you rights and privileges. In return, you must meet the standards of competence, care and conduct set by the GMC.

This booklet sets out the basic principles of good practice. It is not a set of rules, nor is it exhaustive. The GMC publishes more detailed guidance on confidentiality, advertising and the ethical problems surrounding HIV and AIDS

Collins English Dictionary defines principles in terms of standards and vice versa, regarding them as interchangeable in this context. While the introduction denies that the 'principles' to be set out constitute a set of rules, it also states that meeting the standards is a must. At the very least, awareness of what the GMC expect from doctors is a necessary part of medical practice and may help prevent understandings and disputes.

In the 46 paragraphs that follow the headings (Box 13.5) the principles are examined in more detail. A striking feature is the number of times the words (addressed to doctors) 'you must' appear — clearly the GMC takes the principles very seriously; failure to adhere to them could result in the ultimate sanction — suspension or erasure from the medical register and consequent inability to work.

Fitness to practise

The *Medical (Professional Performance) Act* 1995 is the most important extension of the GMC's powers since it was founded in 1858. The GMC has had for years powers to deal with doctors who are unfit to practise because of serious professional misconduct or ill-health; the act has now given it powers to take action against doctors whose standard of professional performance is 'seriously deficient', defined by the GMC as 'a departure from good professional practice', where the standard of a doctor's performance is 'habitually poor'. This may include repeated or persistent failure to comply with the GMC's guidance *Good Medical Practice*, which includes the section *Duties of a Doctor*. The new powers took effect in July 1997, and the performance procedures were implemented in September 1997.

Box 13.5. Duties of a doctor registered with the General Medical Council

Patients must be able to trust doctors with their lives and well-being. To justify that trust, we as a profession have a duty to maintain a good standard of practice and show respect for human life. In particular as a doctor you must:

- Make the care of your patients your first concern
- Treat every patient politely and considerately
- Respect patients' dignity and privacy
- Listen to patients and respect their views
- Respect the right of patients to be fully involved in decisions about their care
- Give patients information in a way that they can understand
- Keep your professional knowledge and skills up to date
- Recognize the limits of your professional competence
- Be honest and trustworthy
- Respect and protect confidential information
- Make sure that your personal beliefs do not prejudice your patients care
- Act quickly to protect patients from risk if you have good reason to believe that you or a colleague may be not be fit to practise
- Avoid abusing your position as a doctor
- Work with colleagues in ways that best serve patients interests

In all these matters, you must never discriminate unfairly against patients or colleagues. And you must always be prepared to justify your actions to them.

The performance procedures
The procedures have four stages (Box 13.6).

Screening
Screening to give initial consideration to complaints which can be made by any member of the public or the medical profession (the paragraph in 'Duties of a Doctor' headed 'Your duty to protect all patients' states 'You must protect patients when you believe that a colleagues conduct, performance or health is a threat to them'. It is now a contractual requirement for doctors to report 'concerns' about the conduct, performance or health of medical colleagues).

Complaints will be referred to one of a team of medical members of the GMC appointed as 'screeners' who will decided if further action is required, and who can request that the doctor undergo an assessment.

Assessment of performance
In which a doctor's practice will be examined in the context of his or her own environment and circumstances by a team of three assessors — two doctors from the relevant specialty and one lay person. The nature of the

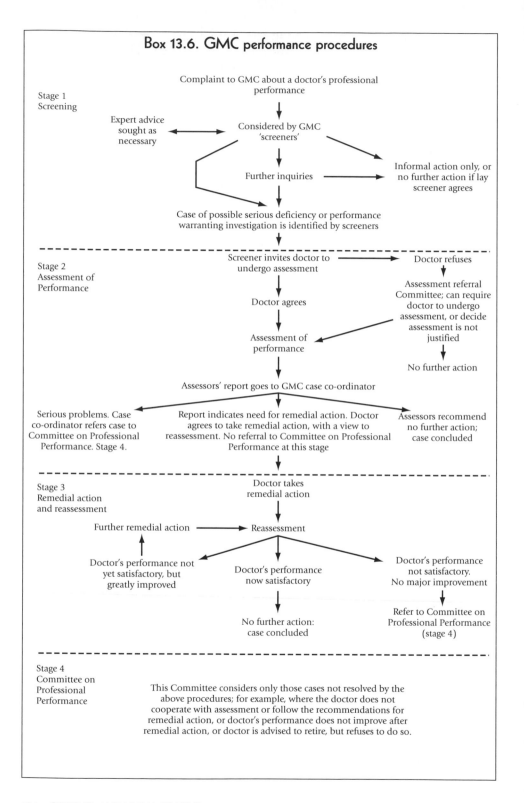

Box 13.6. GMC performance procedures

**Stage 1
Screening**

Complaint to GMC about a doctor's professional performance

Expert advice sought as necessary ⟷ Considered by GMC 'screeners'

Further inquiries ⟶ Informal action only, or no further action if lay screener agrees

Case of possible serious deficiency or performance warranting investigation is identified by screeners

**Stage 2
Assessment of
Performance**

Screener invites doctor to undergo assessment ⟶ Doctor refuses

Assessment referral Committee; can require doctor to undergo assessment, or decide assessment is not justified

Doctor agrees

No further action

Assessment of performance

Assessors' report goes to GMC case co-ordinator

Serious problems. Case co-ordinator refers case to Committee on Professional Performance. Stage 4. ⟵ Report indicates need for remedial action. Doctor agrees to take remedial action, with a view to reassessment. No referral to Committee on Professional Performance at this stage ⟶ Assessors recommend no further action; case concluded

**Stage 3
Remedial action
and reassessment**

Doctor takes remedial action

Further remedial action ⟵ Reassessment

Doctor's performance not yet satisfactory, but greatly improved

Doctor's performance now satisfactory

Doctor's performance not satisfactory. No major improvement

No further action: case concluded

Refer to Committee on Professional Performance (stage 4)

**Stage 4
Committee on
Professional
Performance**

This Committee considers only those cases not resolved by the above procedures; for example, where the doctor does not cooperate with assessment or follow the recommendations for remedial action, or doctor's performance does not improve after remedial action, or doctor is advised to retire, but refuses to do so.

assessment process will probably vary from specialty to specialty, but will be thorough, including a visit to the doctor's workplace, reviews of records, and interviews with the doctor and relevant third parties.

Remedial action and reassessment

The assessors report, if it confirms seriously deficient performance, will lead to the formulation of remedial action, with which the doctor will be invited to participate. The action will vary from case to case and may be supported by post-graduate deans, advisers in general practice or other bodies as appropriate. Reassessment after remedial action will take place, leading, if satisfactory, to no further action, or if unsatisfactory, to referral to the Committee on Professional Performance, a new committee of the GMC established under the new arrangements.

Referral to the Committee on Professional Performance (CPP)

The CPP will determine whether the doctors performance has been seriously deficient. It will normally meet in private, and the doctor and complainant have the right to be present and legally represented. The CPP has statutory powers to impose conditions on, or to withdraw, a doctor's registration.

This procedure has many implications for doctors. Medicine is not an exact science, although increasingly the public believe that scientific and technological advance has made it one. Some problems are difficult, a few impossible to unravel. All treatments have a complications rate and a failure rate. Even in the era of 'evidence-based medicine' there is a range of acceptable treatments for most conditions. When does a 'run' of complications at the hands of say, a surgeon, cease to be a random cluster (one of those things that happen) and become 'a cause for concern' requiring action by colleagues?

A justification stated by the GMC for the new system is that it will encourage doctors to reflect on their practice, examine their standards closely, and consider how they would fare if they were the subject of an assessment. This remains to be seen. At the very least though, a knowledge of what the GMC considers to be *Good Medical Practice* and the duties of a doctor is essential for all doctors throughout their careers.

14. SKILL EXERCISES

These skill exercises are designed to reinforce your knowledge of the topics covered in this book and help you to prepare for job interviews. They do not test the information in this book comprehensively, but reflect the type of questions commonly asked by registrar and consultant interview panels.

1. Getting a job

1. Update your CV and get it checked by your educational supervisor.
2. Arrange for yourself to take part in a mock interview, preferably with video assessment.
3. List the topics that you want to introduce into discussion at your next interview.
4. Write down five topics that you would wish to discuss with a series of applicants for a job in your department. Why did you choose these topics? What answers do you expect from the candidates? What answers would you like? Will answers to these questions help you to discriminate between the candidates?
5. Write down 10 questions you might ask a candidate at an appointments interview. Can you predict the answers they will give (are they closed or semi-closed questions, p. 11)?
6. Attend an appointments interview. Assess what distinguished the successful candidates from those who were not appointed.

3. Organizing yourself

1. Analyse your working week. How much of your time is spent:

- working
- studying
- travelling
- doing things you want to do
- relaxing
- wasted

2. How do these proportions match the type of week that you would like (assuming that you need to earn a salary!). Could you reduce the proportion of time wasted?
3. How many people do you need to communicate with in a day? How much time do you waste trying to contact them? Could you improve efficiency if you or they possessed different means of communication? How many times were you unnecessarily interrupted by a telephone call or bleep?
4. If you lost your diary/organizer, how long would it take you to reproduce the information it contains?

3. Structured training

1. Find out, if you don't know, who are the following people who control your training

   - Your educational supervisor
   - Your post-graduate tutor
   - The college tutor in your chosen speciality
   - The training director in your speciality
   - The regional educational adviser in your speciality
   - The Regional post-graduate dean

   Determine by conversation with senior colleagues what responsibility each of these people has for ensuring that you receive effective training, and how they in turn are supervised.
2. Perform a personal SWOT analysis (p. 123) so that you can judge your strengths and weaknesses. Ask a colleague whom you get on with to perform the same exercise on you from their viewpoint and discuss the results. Ensure that you can still share a pint of beer afterwards!
3. Make sure you understand and can define appraisal and assessment.
4. Update your logbook.

4. Teaching and learning

1. Ask yourself the following questions. How much do you learn by rote? How much do you rely on your memory for retention of fact? How much do you learn from a basis of understanding.
2. Arrange to teach a group of medical students on a topic of mutual interest. List the key items of information that you feel that they should retain at the end of the tutorial. Encourage questions and see which points they have found difficult to comprehend. Arrange to meet them later in the week and discover how much information they have retained.
3. Try writing five MCQ questions. Try them on your colleagues to see whether they find them difficult to understand.

5. Computers and information technology

1. If you do not possess the skills already, consider taking a short course on the basic use of personal computers.
2. Use a typing teacher program to improve your keyboard skills.
3. Read a computer magazine to determine the features of a typical up-to-date personal computer.
4. Discuss with your hospital information department the systems incorporated into your hospital information system to ensure security, back-up of information and disaster resistance. If you have a personal computer, have you taken these aspects into account?

6. Talks and lectures

1. Listen and watch the lecturers at a course and observe how many use repetitive verbal mannerisms, or distracting gestures. Assess the talks using the criteria on pages 71 and 86.
2. Prepare a topic by tape-recording or videoing yourself. Does it sound interesting, do you remain in the centre of the video screen throughout?

7. Visual aids

1. Measure what proportion of transparencies or slides in each lecture were correctly oriented, clean, legible and necessary to the structure of the talk. Which colour scheme did you prefer? Use the criteria on p. 86.
2. Mix the visual aids for your next presentation into a pile; see how quickly you can reassemble them in the correct order and orientation.
3. Produce a single OHT summarizing the main points involved in its production. Project it and note how clearly it can be read from the back of the lecture hall.
4. Use a presentation program to produce the material for your next audit, research or journal club presentation.

8. Quality in medicine

1. Determine what criteria your department has established for the management of emergency patients. In particular, have standards been set for timeliness and skill level of those treating the patients? Do you agree with these standards?
2. Write down the criteria on which you would judge quality in a consumer product — for instance a car.
3. If a relative of yours was admitted with a fractured neck of femur, what care would you want them to receive and what care would you expect them to receive in your own hospital?
4. What systems exist within your clinical service to make sure that action is taken when a positive laboratory result turns up for a patient who has been discharged?
5. Could you explain 'evidence-based medicine' to an interview panel? Can you give an example of how evidence-based medicine affects your daily practice as a clinician?

9. Research

1. Before going to an interview, think of two topics that you think deserve to be researched. Do a literature search to see if there is any existing information on them.
2. Find out if any nearby universities run courses on research methodology and whether you could attend.

3. Write a paragraph trying to explain to a non-medical person a simple technical procedure, for example bladder catheterization. Then give it to a non-medical person and ask them to mark how many words are unfamiliar and whether they understand what the procedure is about.

10. Getting things done

1. What is the role of the 'clinical director' and the 'chairman' of your clinical area. Does one person fill these two posts, or are the roles separate? Who controls the budget?
2. Try to write a 'mission statement' for your department, listing in order of priority the tasks that you think the department should be fulfilling. If your department already has a mission statement compare your effort with the stated aims of the department.
3. Discuss the department budget statement for the past month with the director of the department. Can you make sense of it? How much flexibility does the director have to alter allocations?
4. What improvements would you like to see in your department? What would the implications be, who would they affect and what would they cost?

12. The structure of health care

1. Find out what the contract arrangements are for your department. How easy is it for the department to fulfil these demands?
2. List all the people and departments involved in the care of the next patient you see. (Do not forget to include catering, laundry, stores, secretaries, information department, security, etc.) Decide how you would distribute these costs if you were asked to price the treatment of the patient.
3. Discover what the most expensive drug or piece of disposable equipment used in your clinical service is. Work out how you could save 10% on the cost of this item without affecting the clinical service you offer.

APPENDIX

Further reading

There are only a few easily obtainable books on personal skills which have been written for doctors. Most of our knowledge has come from lectures that we have attended or articles we have read in newspapers, magazines and popular medical journals.

The *How to do it* series from BMJ publishing group contains numerous articles gathered from the regular feature in the *British Medical Journal*. The three volumes add up to over 700 pages and a lot of the information is aimed at established consultants rather than trainees. Some of the articles are quite old. Nevertheless these volumes have contributed to the ideas that we discuss in this book and they are well worth reading.

How to do it. Vols 1–3. BMJ Publishing Group, London 1995.
Each volume costs about £15.

Newble and Cannon's handbook is superb. It uses an unconventional but effective format of type, squiggly lines and cartoons to tell you everything you need to know about teaching and assessment.

David Newble and Robert Cannon, *A Handbook for Medical Teachers*, 3rd Edition, 1994. Kluwer Academic, Lancaster.
Price about £23.

Other suggestions for further reading can be found on pages 63, 90, 143 and 160.

INDEX